BOGS, BATHS
& BASINS

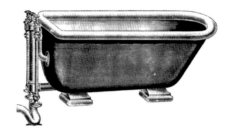

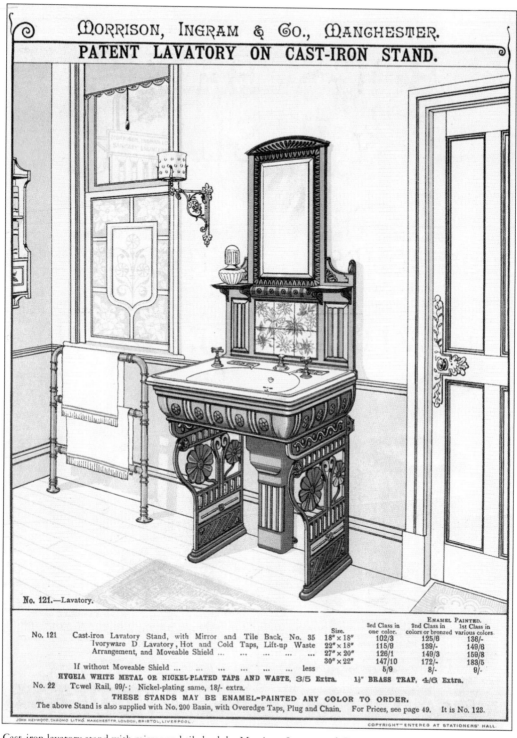

Cast-iron lavatory stand with mirror and tile back by Morrison, Ingram and Co., *c.* 1893. The D-shaped washbasin is supplied with the company's noiseless and steamless taps and a lift-up waste. (*Thomas Crapper and Co. Ltd*)

BOGS, BATHS & BASINS

THE STORY OF
DOMESTIC SANITATION

DAVID J. EVELEIGH

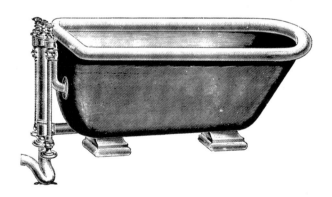

SUTTON PUBLISHING

First published in 2002 by
Sutton Publishing Limited · Phoenix Mill
Thrupp · Stroud · Gloucestershire · GL5 2BU

This paperback edition first published in 2006

British Library Cataloguing in Publication Data
A catalogue record for this book is available from the British Library.

ISBN 0 7509 4125 1

Half-title and title pages: Twyford's Cliffe Vale 'porcelain'-enamelled
fireclay bath, 1898.

Typeset in 11/14pt Garamond.
Typesetting and origination by
Sutton Publishing Limited.
Printed and bound in Great Britain by
J.H. Haynes & Co. Ltd, Sparkford.

To my parents

Contents

Acknowledgements

One of the great pleasures of writing this book has been the extraordinary level of enthusiasm and kindness I have received from so many people. I must start, however, by expressing my deep gratitude to Simon Kirby of Thomas Crapper and Co. and to Terry Wooliscroft at Twyford Bathrooms. Simon and Terry both made valuable comments on the draft text and generously supplied transparencies and photographs from their trade archives. Having the benefit of their profound knowledge of the industry was invaluable. It was also a pleasure to meet Geoffrey Pidgeon who very kindly supplied material and made some valuable observations. It was fascinating talking to Geoffrey, the great-nephew of Frederick Humpherson, who as a young man knew a very elderly George Jennings, the son of Josiah George Jennings – perhaps the greatest sanitary engineer of the nineteenth century.

I am also extremely grateful to Dr Sally Sheard of the Department of Public Health and School of History, at the University of Liverpool, who kindly read some of the text at a busy time and provided details of sanitary conditions in nineteenth-century Liverpool.

I have also received considerable help from colleagues in the museum world. A very big thank you is extended to Roy Brigden and his colleagues, John Creasey, Caroline Benson and Jill Betts at the Rural History Centre, the University of Reading. Roy and John provided access to *The Ironmonger* and other journals while Caroline dealt patiently with my exacting photograph orders. I am also indebted to Ann Eatwell, Assistant Curator in the Metalwork, Silver and Jewellery Department of the Victoria and Albert Museum and her husband Alex Werner, Deputy Head of Later London History and Collections at the Museum of London. They drew many important references to my attention and also provided very comfortable overnight hospitality during some of my research trips to London. At the Russell-Cotes Art Gallery and Museum, Bournemouth, I found a most enthusiastic correspondent in Shaun Garner who provided vital information concerning George Jennings and kindly arranged the photography of the original 'Closet of the Century' in the museum. At the time of writing, a new major gallery of domestic sanitaryware was being created at the Gladstone Pottery Museum, Longton, Stoke-on-Trent, and the Museums Officer, Angela Lee, allowed me to study and photograph some of the exhibits before they went on display. Thanks are also due to Dave Woodcock, Associate Curator of Domestic Technology and Lighting, the Science Museum, Steve Blake, Keeper of Collections, Cheltenham Museum and Art Gallery and to Pam Wooliscroft, Curator of the Spode Museum, Stoke-on-Trent, who very kindly made available some beautiful transparencies of Spode sanitaryware. I would also like to thank Janet Dugdale, Museum of Liverpool Life, Kathy Haslam, Geffrye Museum, Hannah Maddox, Beamish, and Richard de Peyer, Dorset County Museum, for their help.

Elsewhere, I received invaluable assistance from Philip Heath, Heritage Officer for South Derbyshire District Council, concerning the development of sanitaryware manufacture in Swadlincote. Sharpe's Heritage and Arts Trust is currently converting the derelict Sharpe's pottery in Swadlincote into a Heritage and Arts Resource Centre and trust member, Janet Spavold, kindly made available her Master's thesis on the South Derbyshire sanitaryware industry. I am also grateful to James Whitaker of Sharpe Brothers and Co. Ltd who generously allowed me to use illustrations from the company's catalogues. Thanks are also due to Graham Damant, Wimpole Hall, and to the staff of the National Trust Picture Library. I am also grateful to the staff of the British Library, the Public Record Office, the Patent Office, the Science Museum Library, the Wellcome Institute, the Prints and Drawings Department of the British Museum, the Institution of Mechanical Engineers, Brighton Library, Doncaster Library, Manchester Central Library, the Mitchell Library, Glasgow, West Yorkshire Archive Service and the Worshipful Company of Plumbers. I also received fast and efficient service from the National Portrait Gallery's Picture Library, the Bridgeman Art Library and the Mary Evans Picture Library. The picture on page twenty-eight is reproduced by courtesy of the Head of Archives, Staffordshire Record Office. I am also grateful for information supplied by Jo-Ann Buck, John Carnaby, Linda Hall, Helen Hogarth, Nigel Hollingdale, Henry and Joy Moule and Sue Teale. I would also like to thank Michael and Lynn Browning, Steve Hoare and Mary Jane Angell-James for allowing me to photograph their old privies and toilets.

Here in Bristol, I have received help from many quarters. I am extremely grateful to Sir George White for providing photographs of his great-grandfather's luxurious bathroom, of 1900, and also, in his capacity as Curator of The Worshipful Company of Clockmakers, going to some considerable trouble to photograph a portrait of Alexander Cummings in the possession of the company. I also received help and enthusiastic encouragement from Bob Chambers at Bristol Water. Thanks are also due to Jonathan Erskine, Avon Archaeological Unit, and the staff of the Central Reference Library, Bristol, and in particular, Anthony Beeson. I also received friendly help from John Williams, the City Archivist, and his colleagues, particularly Richard Burley and Alison Brown. I am also grateful to Melissa Barnett for lending me her precious original copy of Mayhew. I must thank Ray Barnett, the Collections Manager, at Bristol City Museum and Art Gallery, for his quiet support, without which this book might not have been possible. Many colleagues have chipped in with help and advice including Gail Boyle, Roger Clark, Andy Cotton, Jeremy Dixon, Sue Giles, Kate Newnham, Sarah Riddle, Gareth Salway, Sheena Stoddard and Karin Walton. Finally, special thanks are due to Alison Crawford, the Assistant Curator of Social History, at Blaise Castle House Museum, who read much of the text and made many suggestions to ensure it was intelligible. Moreover, she has put up with me talking virtually non-stop about toilets and other sanitary appliances for the last eighteen months with amazing patience!

Many others have written to me over the past few years with their recollections of old privies and lecturing around the country for the National Association of Decorative and Fine Arts and other organisations; I have met many people who have taken the trouble to pass information on to me. To all of you, I am most grateful.

David J. Eveleigh
Bristol, March 2002

Introduction

Walk around any historic house open to the public and on a busy day you will see visitors impressed by the scale and grandeur of the furnishings – the state beds, the large gilt mirrors and chandeliers. But the question that is often on their lips as they file through the rooms is, how did the former occupants of the house go to the toilet? Or, did they wash, and if so, how? As a museum curator specialising in domestic history, I am frequently quizzed about the 'invention' of the modern toilet and sometimes, people take me to one side and with a nod and wink begin to tell me about Thomas Crapper.

These are not easily answered questions. The development of our present-day sanitary appliances – the water closet or toilet, the bath and the washbasin – and of the bathroom itself – has received surprisingly little attention. With a few commendable exceptions, books on domestic architecture and interiors generally have little to say on the subject. A few specialist studies have appeared, such as Lawrence Wright's *Clean and Decent* first published in 1960. Then in 1978, Lucinda Lambton brought the genius of the art of the late Victorian sanitaryware potter to a wider audience in a beautifully illustrated book, *Temples of Convenience*. More recently, the television presenter Adam Hart-Davis has produced an informative and entertaining A to Z of toilet facts, *Thunder, Flush and Thomas Crapper*. Thanks to him, we now know how an astronaut deals with those unavoidable 'calls of nature' in zero gravity. Yet much of the detail of how and when particular types of fittings were introduced has remained virgin territory for the researcher.

The paradox is that fascination with the subject has long been tempered by a natural reluctance to probe the details of such a private and personal subject. The taboo which surrounds the act of defecation – and to a lesser extent, urination – has extended to the equipment, and thus limited our understanding of this important area of domestic history. Victorian ladies were, by all accounts, capable of blushing at the sight of water closets on display in a sanitary engineer's showroom. Today, the public is less likely to offer a toilet to a museum than a disused mangle, gas cooker or sewing machine. After all, it is difficult to be proud of a dirty old toilet!

Similarly, literary references to personal habits and matters of hygiene are hard to come by. There are exceptions, of course: Samuel Pepys, the seventeenth-century diarist is obligingly frank on the subject, but then he is on most things. A few autobiographical accounts of Victorian country life briefly describe the simple sanitary arrangements which generally prevailed. Edwin Grey (b. *c.* 1860), who spent his childhood in rural Hertfordshire in the late 1860s and 1870s, describes the shared privies in his village, and Flora Thompson (1876–1947), writing of life in a north Oxfordshire hamlet in the 1880s, unusually describes how cottage families washed. But one searches in vain for references in novels. The characters who populate the works of Charles Dickens, Emily Brontë and Thomas Hardy, for example, light fires, fill kettles, cook, smoke pipes and extinguish lamps and candles, but never go to the toilet, wash or take a bath. The same reticence on such matters also restricts the visual record. While beautiful women, reclining dreamily in baths, have made socially acceptable subjects for the artist, representations of people sitting on closets are confined to the ribald and satirical cartoon. So we have 'Sawney', the unsophisticated High-lander, jumping feet first into a London bog in 1745 and 'Milord Plumpudding' staring stupidly at us as he sits on a commode after gorging himself on a huge meal of meat, pies and red wine.

The subject can indeed be amusing, but it does, nevertheless, merit serious attention, and this book is intended to provide a detailed account of how our modern bathroom fittings have evolved. Making fittings that made homes cleaner, healthier and more comfortable was clearly the chief impulse behind the development of sanitaryware, and so this book is chiefly concerned with progress in the home. The book also explains how the creation of fitted baths and washbasins led to the widespread adoption of bathrooms from the late nineteenth century. For most people, this was an entirely new room which raised new questions concerning its furnishing and decorative treatment. Public facilities – in the street, in public buildings such as the Crystal Palace and in institutions – raised different issues, some of which influenced the mainstream development of sanitaryware. But this book is not concerned with the detail of the provision of public toilets and urinals, or the design of toilet facilities for ships or railway coaches. Equally, it has to be acknowledged that the field of sanitaryware technology is wider than domestic fittings alone. Some of the leading manufacturers – notably Doulton – made drainpipes and a wide range of hardware connected with house and street and drainage. But this is primarily a book about domestic appliances, although even within the confines of the home it is not a story for the faint hearted.

Notwithstanding the elusive and private nature of the subject, there are still, many sources available which enable us to build up a picture of how domestic sanitary appliances evolved. Technical information from the inventors and manufacturers exists in the form of patents and trade literature. In the late nineteenth century lavishly illustrated trade catalogues were published by a wide range of manufacturers. Sanitary engineers were no exception, and some of the colour plates in catalogues of the 1880s and 1890s – a few are reproduced here in colour – emphasise the beauty of many domestic sanitary fittings of this period. The catalogues also provide vital clues concerning the introduction of new models and their claimed advantages. Reviews of new inventions and advertisements also appear in professional and trade journals such as *The Builder* and *The Ironmonger*. Builders'

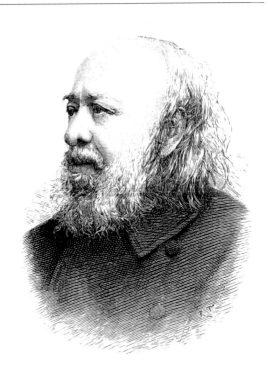

Edwin Chadwick (1800–90).

manuals and encyclopaedias of domestic economy provide useful surveys and appraisals of the range of sanitary appliances available, and from the 1870s, an increasing number of specialist books concerning sanitation and hygiene appeared. Many of these also contain comprehensive reviews of the equipment.

There is also a huge body of evidence about sanitary arrangements contained in the official reports, in particular those concerned with public health. The public health movement and the spread of the sanitary idea provided the impetus for the revolution in standards of domestic sanitation which occurred in the nineteenth century. Edwin Chadwick (1800–90) stands as a colossus over the movement. In the 1830s from the reports he received as Secretary to the Poor Law Commission, he came to see that insanitary conditions bred disease. But he was no sentimentalist. He wanted to end the waste and expense that fevers and other diseases caused. His Report into the Sanitary Condition of the Labouring Population of Great Britain, published in 1842, revealed the extent of the insanitary and overcrowded conditions of the poor districts in large towns across the country. Further reports compiled by the Health of Towns Commission and the Board of Health, which Chadwick chaired, only served to show how widespread the problem was. The *laissez-faire* – or do nothing – approach of previous governments which had allowed these problems to expand in direct proportion to the expansion of the urban population, was overturned by a realisation that legislation had to be introduced if physical conditions for the labouring population were to improve. Chadwick appreciated, above all, that the health and comfort of civilised society in towns depended on establishing arrangements for bringing water in and wastes out: that is, providing constant piped water, mains sewers and house drains. Without the solutions to these problems which were created, largely as a direct consequence of public-health reform, the general adoption of the bathroom and its fittings could never have taken place.

There was, therefore, an obvious social dimension to public-health reform. The scarcity of adequate sanitary arrangements in the poorer districts of towns pointed to the absence of law and order among the inhabitants. If cleanliness was next to Godliness, filth and dirt suggested moral depravity and perhaps even represented a threat to the social order. This undercurrent to public-health reform shaped the measures devised by public-health reformers – a loose alliance of politicians, medical doctors and clergymen, engineers, progressive architects and the growing band of sanitary manufacturers. Their investigations convinced them of the inability of the poor to keep themselves clean and so they introduced sanitary reforms – and new sanitary appliances – which only served to underline class divisions.

Disposing of human excrement safely and economically was the overriding concern from the 1840s. In some towns, the solution was to effectively restrict the use of water closets to a privileged few, while various kinds of dry closets involving the use of ash, earth and buckets were introduced for use by the poor. Where the use of water closets was adopted more generally, class distinctions were still only too apparent. Working-class water closets were usually placed outside houses in backyards or in back lanes and were of distinct types. There were simple and cheap closets for use by servants and cottage dwellers and in the crowded courts of some northern towns, communal trough closets were installed. Many sanitary appliances intended for use by the working classes were designed upon the assumption that they were incapable of flushing their own closets! The result was a plethora of inventions for self-acting or automatic devices. The dictum of many sanitary reformers could well have been 'simple closets for simple folk'.

As Victorian legislation placed much of the responsibility – and authority – for sanitary reform in the hands of local authorities, the result was the development of a staggering variety of sanitary appliances. While many middle-class villas and large houses across the country had their expensive valve closets, most industrial towns in the Midlands and the north devised their own distinctive systems. In the 1870s, a visitor to the poorer parts of Leeds, Liverpool and

Birkenhead would have found trough or tumbler closets in general use, while parts of Manchester and Salford were provided with semi-automatic ash closets. Rochdale had its tubs and Halifax its padded pails. There were also striking contrasts to be found in the countryside – between well-ordered estates where well-maintained earth closets were supplied for the tenants and the squalor which prevailed, for example, in parts of west Cornwall. Such diversity of arrangements disappeared in the twentieth century, and at the beginning of the twenty-first is hard to imagine. But one of the strange twists in the technological development outlined in this book is that the modern 'loo' was developed out of some of the simpler water closets intended for use by people in humble circumstances – and not the expensive and sophisticated closets used by the well-to-do.

When it came to other aspects of personal hygiene – washing and taking a bath – the same class divisions were evident. While bathing became an established part of middle-class life in the middle decades of the nineteenth century, the solution for the working classes was to provide public bath houses. The principle of including baths with running hot and cold water in working-class homes was only en-shrined in legislation after 1918. And some older houses had to wait until the 1950s and 1960s before they acquired their first fitted bath.

Having the use of an indoor toilet and bathroom is now an essential component of civilised life across much of the English-speaking world. Civilisation and sanitation have been inseparable to public-health reformers and sanitary engineers alike since the nineteenth century. The makers Shanks, in their catalogue for 1930, wrote, 'one index of advancing civilisation is the importance that is now being attached to the installation of bathrooms'. Many writers looked back to a 'golden age' of the Romans who, as town dwellers, had been confronted by the same issues and had devised their own sanitary arrangements. They introduced main sewers in streets, organised the supply of water, built public baths and even devised closets supplied with water. The discovery of these facilities in well-preserved Roman towns such as Pompeii was contrasted with the virtual absence of any equivalent in mid-Victorian Britain. When bathroom suites were first made in the 1880s, some were dressed up in the 'Roman' or 'Pompeian' style. Sanitation, therefore, has ancient antecedents and even predates the Romans by several millennia. Remains of privies in the palace of the Sumerian king, Sargon – over 4,000 years old – have been uncovered, and closets connected to drains almost 5,000 years old have been found at Mohenjo-Daro in India.

Nevertheless, the book does not attempt a chronological account of sanitation from the world's earliest civilisations to the present day.

This story is chiefly concerned with the period of development which began slowly in the late eighteenth century and then gathered momentum during the nineteenth century. It reached a peak in the 1870s and 1880s when, in a matter of a few years, the basic principles governing the design of present-day water closets, baths and washbasins were established. This represented a major British technological achievement (the American sanitaryware industry only began to find its feet in the 1890s), and considering its importance to the quality of our lives today remains one that has been sadly neglected by historians. Whilst the engineers who produced the steam ship and the railway locomotive are known to us, those who perfected sanitary equipment have been lost in obscurity. How many people, for example, are familiar with the name of Josiah George Jennings, arguably the greatest sanitary engineer of the nineteenth century? Jennings was not alone: Henry Doulton, John Shanks and Thomas W. Twyford also played a major part in improving sanitary equipment after 1850. There were others, too, who made lasting contributions. Edmund Sharpe, for example, a Swadlincote potter – the first to patent a flushing rim for water closets – and Frederick Humpherson, who produced the first pedestal wash-down water closet, made in one piece of ceramicware; this was to become the most widely used water closet of the twentieth century. Humpherson had learned his trade as an apprentice of Thomas Crapper in Chelsea. Crapper has achieved almost mythical status as an inventor of water closets, but in reality, he is representative of the many self-made men who brought wealth to themselves and to the country by establishing an important manufacturing industry. And probably everyone who reads this book will be grateful that our lives came after and not before theirs.

CHAPTER ONE

Loathsomeness and Indecency
privy-middens, close stools and chamber pots

Recent excavations at Yorvik, the Viking settlement at York, uncovered a 1,000-year-old 'toilet' seat. It consists of a simple wooden board – forming a bench – with a round hole cut out.[1] The seat would have once covered a void where human excrement would have piled up. Instantaneous removal of the waste, by gravity or running water, was rather the exception. This basic facility continued in use, little changed, into the twentieth century. Many still survive in situ, albeit mostly disused. They would be instantly recognisable to a tenth-century Norse settler – or anyone for that matter – living in Britain at the time. This simple arrangement, nevertheless, varied enormously in detail and went by many names. Parson Woodforde (1740–1803), the eighteenth-century diarist, called his the 'jericho'. The 'necessary' was another common term, so was 'closet' and 'privy' – or 'privy-midden' – the midden being the pile of dung. And there was 'bog' but never 'toilet'. The association of the words 'toilet' and 'lavatory' with a device for the removal of human waste is modern and appears to date from the early twentieth century. Formerly toilet meant the act of washing and dressing or it referred to a dressing table with a mirror. Toilet-ware denoted the utensils which went with it – sets of ewers or jugs and washbasins and the lavatory was properly the washbasin.

A further confusion is the use of some names to describe both the actual device, with its wooden seat and the room or space where it was located. Sometimes a distinction was made by adding the word 'house', as in 'bog house' and 'necessary house'. Many were separate from the dwelling although in larger houses it was common for them to be incorporated within the main building. Medieval castles were often provided with garderobes in upper floors which conveyed the waste by stone chutes built in the thickness of the walls to the surrounding moat or ditch. At Conway Castle in North Wales, built between 1283 and 1293, some of the privies consist of corbelled projections overhanging the rock below.[2] A south wing added to Little Moreton Hall, near Congleton in Cheshire, between 1570 and 1580 includes a garderobe tower containing two first-floor closets which emptied through holes in the bottom of the cess chamber into the moat.[3] Similar projecting turrets connecting with first-floor chambers were frequently built into the walls of substantial farmhouses of the sixteenth and seventeenth centuries. A draft specification of 1724 for a 50 ft wide town house alongside the quay in the centre of Bristol includes four chambers on the 'Best Chamber Floor'. Three of them had closets which, 'will be of great convenience for the holding of close stools and many other family necessaries'.[4]

Close stools were essentially portable privies with a soil pan enclosed in a box-like stool. A hinged lid covered the seat which contained a round hole. Surviving examples are rare, although two sumptuous examples with padded seats and covered in red velvet survive at Hampton Court and Knole near Sevenoaks – the latter was apparently used by James II (1633–1701, r. 1685–88).[5] Close stools were also covered in leather and are occasionally listed in household inventories dating from the seventeenth and eighteenth centuries. An inventory of the furnishings of Hardwick Hall, Derbyshire, attached to the will of Arabella Stuart (1575–1615), made in 1601, lists several leather close stools in the chambers or in adjoining closets. Within her own bed chamber there was an inner room containing 'a close stoole covered with blewe cloth stitcht with white, with red and black silk frenge'. There were three pewter basins so that a fresh one was always in place while the others were being emptied.[6] They were also used lower down the social scale: John Durrell, a carpenter of Dawley in Shropshire, left a 'close stool and pan in the chamber over the parlour' when he died in 1728.[7]

Chamber pots were also widely used. They are listed in 24 out of 248 farmhouse and cottage inventories covering the period 1635 to 1749 from Writtle in mid-Essex.[8] Archaeological excavations of sixteenth and seventeenth-century sites confirm that many were made of brown earthenware, although more valuable – and durable – pewter chamber pots were also common: 11 of those listed in the Writtle inventories were made of pewter. The 1682 inventory of Thomas Hitchen, a farmer in Wellington, Shropshire records two

'And so to bed, and in the night was mightely troubled by a looseness . . . and so I was forced in this strange house to rise and shit in the chimney . . .'
Samuel Pepys, 1665.

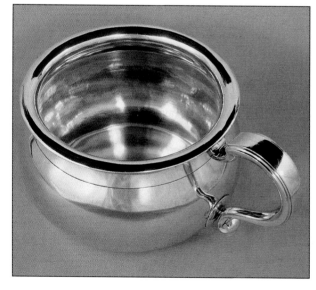

A silver chamber pot by the London silversmith, Daniel Piers, 1747, from Dunham Massey, Cheshire. (*National Trust*)

pewter chamber pots valued together at 1s.[9] More rarely they were made of sheet brass, and for a small elite of royal or aristocratic users, there were chamber pots of silver. In the eighteenth century, chamber pots were also made of tin-glazed earthenware (delftware) and porcelain, and by the later part of the century in white earthenware. In the nineteenth century, a vast range of decorated earthenware chamber pots was produced. Humour entered the chamber pot. Some contained a portrait of Napoleon and others humorous verses: thus, 'use me well and keep me clean and I'll not tell what I've seen'.

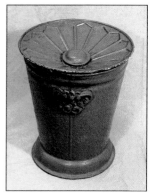

Nineteenth-century tinplate slop bucket, from Clevedon Court, Somerset.

At Hardwick Hall, Derbyshire, in 1601, chamber pots were found beside the close stool, suggesting they were used primarily for urine, although owing to the candour of Samuel Pepys (1633–1703) we know that this was not always the case. In September 1665 he wrote, '. . . and so to bed and in the night was mightely troubled with a looseness (I suppose from some fresh damp linen that I put on this night) and feeling for a chamber pot, there was none, I having called the mayde up out of her bed, she had forgot I suppose to put one there; so I was forced in this strange house to rise and shit in the chimney twice; and so to bed and was very well again.'[10] It was important for some that the chamber pot was not only to hand but also clean. Travelling through Germany in the summer of 1767, Lady Mary Coke (1726–1811) wrote, 'I have bought more china and among other things a chamber pot. I have found such dirty ones upon the road that it will be of use to me all my journey.'[11]

In larger houses servants would deal with the chamber pots, delivering them to bed chambers in the evening and emptying them in the morning. In the nineteenth century, specially made slop buckets were used by servants to carry away the contents. These tinplate vessels had funnel-like lids with a central hole covered by a small dome. Chamber pots, of course, were often placed under the bed, although eighteenth-century cabinet makers, such as Thomas Chippendale (1718–79) and George Hepplewhite (d. 1786), supplied designs for fashionable night tables or pot cupboards for the storage of chamber pots. Among eighteenth-century 'polite' society, chamber pots were also available in dining rooms where they were kept in sideboards made with a pot cupboard at the back or side. The chamber pot could then be used by men once the ladies had withdrawn. Foreign visitors were disgusted at the open and casual manner in which the chamber pot was used in view of the company. As a guest of an English family in Suffolk in 1784, François de la Rochefoucauld (1765–1848), a young Frenchman, described how 'the sideboard is garnished also with chamber pots in line with the common practice of going over to the sideboard to pee, while the others are drinking. Nothing is hidden. I find that very indecent'.[12]

'I have bought more china and among other things a chamber pot. I have found such dirty ones upon the road that it will be of use to me all my journey.' Lady Mary Coke in Frankfurt, 1767.

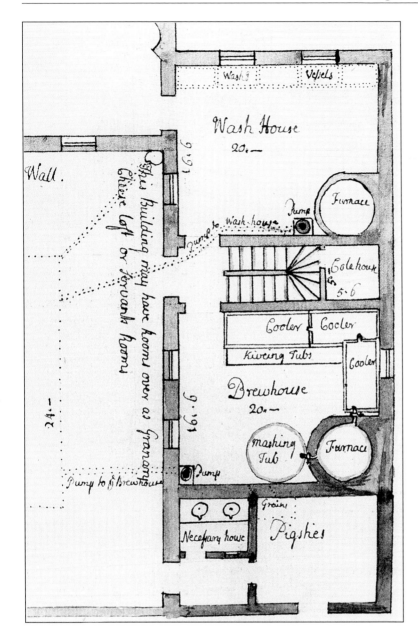

A plan of a service wing of a large house showing the 'necessary house' next to the pigsties and alarmingly close to the water pump. From Sir John Vanbrugh's designs for Kings Weston, Gloucestershire, *c.* 1720. (*Bristol Record Office*)

Built-in privies were often placed at ground or even basement level where they were sited directly over a midden – a pit or cesspool – where the waste was allowed to accumulate. In the mid-1840s, Henry Austin, the secretary to the Health of Towns Association, visited Worcester where he found houses in the High Street with 'necessaries' in the cellars. The consequences were appalling. They were difficult to empty and, moreover, 'offensive effluvium' was, according to Austin, 'perpetually poisoning the atmosphere in the houses'.[13] Privies were better placed at the far end of houses where the emptying caused less

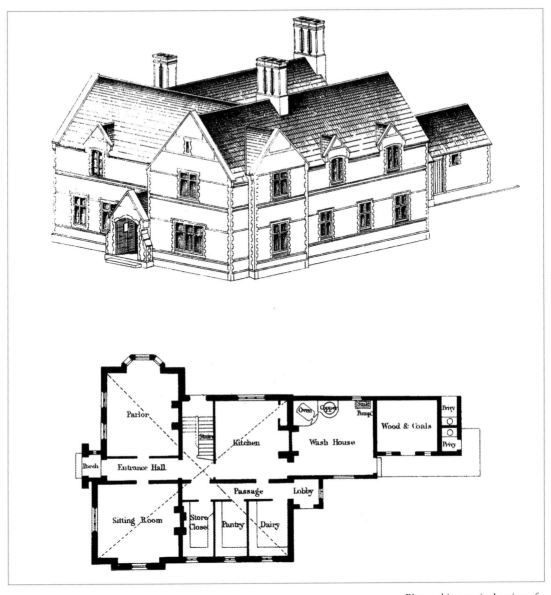

Plan and isometric drawing of a farm house, *c*. 1850, erected by W. Hans Sloane Stanley at Rollestone near Southampton. The service wing is at the back of the house and contains a privy in a single-storey extension at the far end beyond the wood and coal store. The six-bedroom house, of course, at this date had no bathroom. From J. Bailey Denton, *The Homesteads of England*, 1855.

disruption to the household. In large houses they were sometimes added to the end of a ground-floor service wing. Plans for a service block at Kings Weston House, south Gloucestershire, from about 1720 attributed to Sir John Vanbrugh (1664–1726) show a 'necessary house', a small structure behind the brewhouse and next to the pig sty.[14] Large, well-appointed farmhouses illustrated in J. Bailey Denton's *The Farm Homesteads of England*, from 1855, in most cases show a similar arrangement with privies housed in a single-storeyed extension at the rear of the service wing or behind livestock sheds and reached by a separate external door.

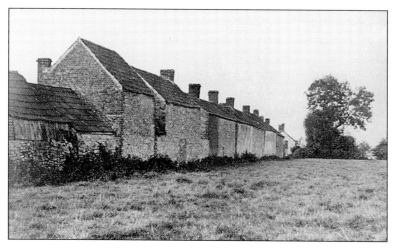

The rear of cottages in Somerset, built on a narrow strip of land between the road and fields. There were no gardens front or back and no space, therefore, to build separate privies. Instead they were wedged in small sheds between the houses. They had formerly consisted of 'offensive privies', but by the time this photograph was taken, in about 1914, they had been converted to pail closets.

Many privies, however, consisted of separate structures, detached from the house. In towns they were often found in backyards – this was the 'bog house' of eighteenth-century London[15] – and in the countryside, they were usually located in back gardens, as far from the house as possible. In her account of life in a north Oxfordshire hamlet in the 1880s, Flora Thompson describes the privy as a 'little beehive-shaped building at the bottom of the garden or in a corner of the wood and tool shed known as the hovel'. She also recalled the irritation of having to walk half-way down the garden under an umbrella in wet weather to reach the closet.[16] When the journey had to be made in the dark, lanterns (or in the twentieth century, torches) were carried to light the way. The structures varied considerably. Some were all-wooden shacks. The making of these and their seats by a specialist carpenter is described in laconic style by Charles Sale in a book originally published in America in 1929.[17] Many, of course, like the main house were built of stone which varied according to the local geology. Some were of brick. Roofs were sometimes double pitched which created a picturesque front to the structure with the door centred below a gable in miniature, but many had the simpler and cheaper single-pitched roof. In 1915, William Savage, a medical officer of health in Somerset, said, 'often they are very deplorable structures'.[18]

But sometimes there was no privy at all. Facilities had to be shared by several households. Describing life in a Hertfordshire village in the late 1860s and 1870s, Edwin Grey remarked how the privies were anything but private, some having to serve as many as six cottages.[19] As late as 1912, it was reported that in the parish of Port Isaac, Cornwall, sixty-four houses out of ninety inspected had no closet accommodation of any kind.[20] Heavily used and with no one taking responsibility for cleaning or emptying them, shared privies were usually the very worst. In Worcester, Henry Austin came across

'There's a lot of fine points to putting up a first class privy that the average man don't think about.'
'Lem Putt', *The Specialist*, 1929.

a necessary which was used by more than fifteen families. This, he wrote, 'presented to me one of the most horrible examples of loathsomeness and indecency that it has ever been my lot, with some experiences of such matters to witness. I will not sicken you,' he added, 'with details of these horrible scenes.'[21]

Privies were mostly one-room structures. The walls were usually white-washed or painted in various pastel shades – yellow ochre, pink or blue – the latter frequently used in kitchens because it was believed to be repellent to flies. Simple wooden panelling sometimes lined the wall a foot or two above the seat. Printed material, verses or pictures sometimes decorated the walls. The London bog house visited by 'Sawney', the fictitious Highlander lampooned, it is believed, by William Hogarth (1697–1764) in 1745, is covered with various ballads and verses. The privies of the 1880s recalled by Flora Thompson were similarly adorned with pictures from periodicals: scenes such as the bombardment of Alexandria or the Tay Bridge

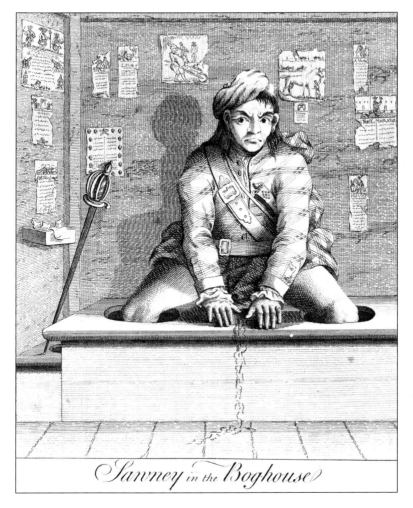

Sawney in the Boghouse

Sawney in a London Bog House, 1745. This satirical print, attributed to Hogarth, pokes fun at Sawney, the primitive Highlander, who had never seen a privy or bog hole until he visited London. Upon being shown to the bog house he 'thrusts his brawney thighs down the two holes, And squeezing, cry'd – "Sawney's a Laird, I trow Neer did he naably disembaage 'till now".' Note the child's seat to the left and the printed matter pinned to the wall. (*British Museum*)

Disaster, which showed the end of the train
dangling from the broken bridge. Portraits of
political leaders were also popular: Gladstone,
Lord Salisbury or Lord Randolph Churchill
depending, of course, on political allegiances.
Sometimes health or sanitary maxims were
chalked or pencilled on the walls. Otherwise,
the interiors were plain with perhaps a simple
recess in the wall to take a candle or lantern.
Flora Thompson also recalled that 'privies
were as good an index as any to the characters
of their owners. Some were horrible holes;
others were fairly decent with the seat
scrubbed to snow whiteness and the brick
floor raddled.'[22]

Surviving seats are often made of deal,
although it is likely that before the nineteenth century many were made of elm. They
often filled the entire back wall of the privy,
and frequently contained more than one hole.
Two-hole seats with one opening larger than
the other were common, but occasionally
three or more holes were provided. They were
often spacious. The seat of a disused privy in

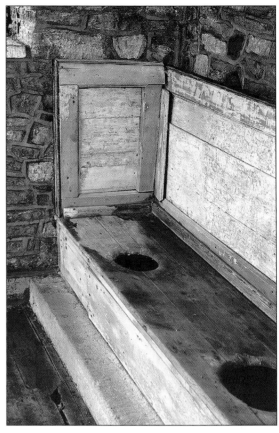

the back garden of a house in Hallatrow, Somerset, is 10 ft wide and
contains three holes. The smallest has just a diameter of 7 in, the
largest in the centre is 10 in, while the right-hand one is just a ½ in
smaller. Small holes were obviously for children and were sometimes
set lower. Four- or even six-hole seats were rare but have been
recorded, and some larger ones filled two walls. The holes were either
round or oval and were usually covered with detachable lids which
helped keep smells in and insects out. The lids were usually round
themselves with turned wooden knobs, battens or finger holes. Most
that survive are of deal or pine like the seat, but the lids of the three-
hole privy at Hallatrow are made of elm and are hexagonal in shape.
The use of seats with two or more holes suggests that using a privy
was not necessarily a solitary activity. Children, at least, would use
them together and the three-hole privy at Hallatrow was used by a
family of thirteen until 1910. Every evening the eleven children
would walk across the back garden using a candle on dark evenings
to use the privy before going to bed, the older children doubtless
using the adult-sized holes.

The arrangement under the seat varied. While the majority of
privies were placed over a pit some were located over running water

A three-hole privy at Elm Tree
Farm, Hallatrow, Somerset.
The seat is 10 ft wide and
contains three holes, graded in
size. The smallest, seen here on
the left, has a diameter of 7 in
and was obviously for children.
The centre one seen on the
right is the largest with a
diameter of 10 in, while the
right-hand hole, out of view,
has a diameter of 9½ in. The
privy was last used by the
Harrison family, consisting of
John Harrison, his wife, Ann,
and their fourteen children
between 1850 and 1910.

in order that the waste would be washed away. Francis George Heath found cottages at Wrington, Somerset, in about 1880 where the closets were built over the village brook although, unfortunately, the villagers also drew some of their water supply from the same brook.[23] A similar arrangement remained in use in the first half of the twentieth century at Highridge Farm, Dundry in north Somerset, where the privy consisted of a small limestone structure built over a brick-arched culvert supplied with water from an underground stream. The flow of water varied from a small trickle during a dry summer to a raging torrent after heavy rain. In towns, privies were found overhanging the rivers. Ramshackle wooden privies lined the open stretches of the River Fleet in London until covered over in the 1840s, and in Bristol similar structures overhung the muddy banks of the River Frome on its course through the centre of the city. The waste was only washed away at times of particularly high tides: in 1844, a local doctor, Dr William Budd (1811–80) reported, 'the state of things in the interval is too loathsome and disgusting to describe'.[24]

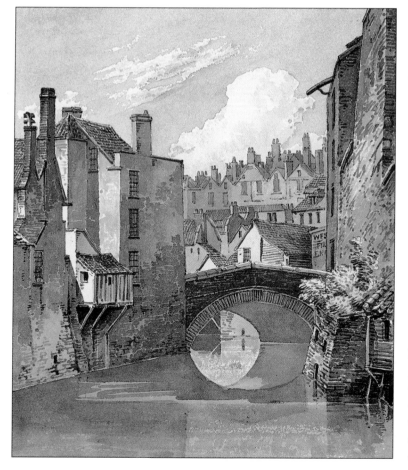

The River Frome flowing under St John's Bridge in the centre of Bristol looks attractive enough in this watercolour of 1821 by Hugh O'Neill, but in 1845 it was described as the city's worst sewage nuisance. Raw sewage drained into the river and ramshackle privies that hung directly over the river deposited their filth on to the muddy banks of the river directly underneath. Perhaps, not surprisingly, O'Neill has painted the scene at high tide! These privies and most of the houses with them disappeared between 1857 and 1867 when the course of the Frome through the city was covered over. (*Bristol City Museum and Art Gallery*)

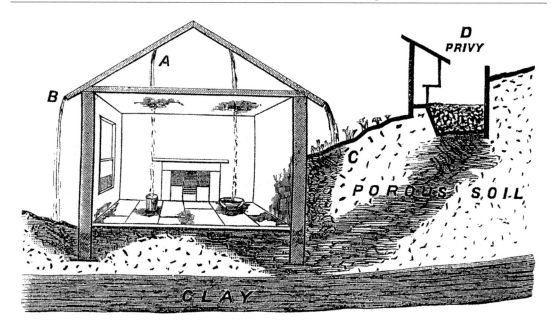

The typical privy, however, possessed no means for disposing of waste and was, in effect, a storehouse of excrement: a pile of dung – the midden – being an essential component. Sometimes the catchment was simply the bare earth beneath the seat, but many privies were built over a large vault or deep pit that extended beyond the back of the structure. The pits or cesspools varied in depth, shape and the nature of the lining – if there was one – moreover, they varied from one part of the country to another. In early Victorian London, Henry Mayhew (1812–87), the author of *London Labour and the London Poor*, distinguished between two kinds of older cesspools found in the metropolis. Soil tanks were the 'filth receptacles' of larger houses. They varied in size, but according to Mayhew, some were deep and well made in solid masonry. 'Bog holes' consisted of a hole dug into the earth with less masonry than a soil tank and sometimes with none at all. Again they varied in shape and size: some were round, others oblong and on average contained a cubic yard of matter. Occasionally, two or more bog holes drained into a soil tank placed in 'an obscure part of the garden or backyard'. Bog holes were rarely watertight and this was usually intentional – so that the liquid portion of the sewage could drain away – reducing its bulk and postponing the removal.[25] In some towns – Northampton, Guildford, Leicester and Bridport, for example – the underlying strata was sufficiently porous for the cesspools to drain freely into the ground so that emptying was not required. At Steyning in Sussex, they drained into open ditches and at Penzance, after a heavy shower, into the gutters.[26]

A diagram, published in 1892, representing a dilapidated and insanitary cottage built into a hillside. The privy-midden consists of a separate structure above the level of the ground floor with the seat directly above the pit which is dug into porous soil allowing the liquid sewage to contaminate the surrounding land.

Leaking and overflowing cesspools represented a major threat to health. Seeping liquid sewage running through porous soil could contaminate nearby wells, spreading diseases such as cholera, typhoid and diarrhoea. In such cases, according to George Wilson in 1873, the soil around wells was often sodden with soakage from privies. In consequence, people lived, 'in an atmosphere charged with the . . . gases given off by the decomposition of their own excrement' while they drank 'water tainted by the foul liquid which oozes from the excremental mass'.[27] Cholera was the new killer disease of mid-nineteenth-century Britain. It had first appeared in 1831 and over the next four decades, many thousands died in major epidemics in London and other large towns. Capable of killing victims within hours and spreading with deadly speed, the nature of the disease was the source of wild speculation among the medical profession, its causes a mystery. The 'miasma' or atmospheric theory – that disease was carried in bad air – was then the accepted orthodoxy. 'All smell is disease,' claimed Edwin Chadwick, the great sanitary reformer, in 1846, and two years earlier, one of his close associates, Dr Neil Arnott (1788–1874), had stated that the cause of many diseases was the 'poison of atmospheric impurity'. Chadwick and his supporters were keen to see privies and cesspools removed – not because of the risk of contamination to water – but to the atmosphere. The danger posed by privy-middens to water supplies was only gradually recognised from the 1850s as the evidence for the water-borne nature of cholera increased.

Regular emptying of cesspools was often required, although it was sometimes neglected, as Samuel Pepys discovered in 1660. 'Going down to my cellar,' he wrote on 20 October, 'I put my foot into a great heap of turds, by which I find that Mr Turner's house of office is full and comes into my cellar.'[28] Clearly, the amount of emptying depended on the size of the pit, the frequency of its use and the quality of the lining. The cesspools in Flora Thompson's north Oxfordshire hamlet were emptied twice yearly, while in London Mayhew said it was done once every two years. It was not a pleasant occurrence: the stench was intolerable and the doors and windows of neighbouring houses were kept firmly shut. Also, it was usually carried out after dark by nightmen who worked by lantern light. In early Victorian London, the legal hours for nightwork were between midnight and five in the morning.[29] In large towns and cities, the removal of the waste was big business. Some contractors were men of capital – 'well to do in the world', according to Mayhew – owning a considerable number of horses and carts and employing a large workforce. Mayhew's research in London revealed that nightwork was not a 'distinct calling'. The master nightmen, he found, were 'generally master chimney sweepers, scavengers, rubbish carters and builders'.[30] The labourers were likewise drawn from other trades. 'The generality of nightmen', Mayhew said, 'are scavengers, or dustmen, or chimney sweepers, or rubbish carters, or pipe layers, or ground workers or coal porters, carmen or stablemen, or men working for the market gardeners round London – all either in or out of employment.'[31]

Thanks to Mayhew's investigative skills we have a vivid and detailed picture of how nightmen went about their work. Some cesspools were emptied by the 'hydraulic method', using pumps and hose to convey the waste to the nearest sewer but most were emptied manually using shovels, scoops and tubs. Late one evening, Mayhew went to see a gang at work. Large horn lanterns were placed at the edge of the cesspool to illuminate the scene and in the still of the night, the men began their work. A typical gang consisted of four labourers: one, the 'holeman', would stir the refuse to loosen it and

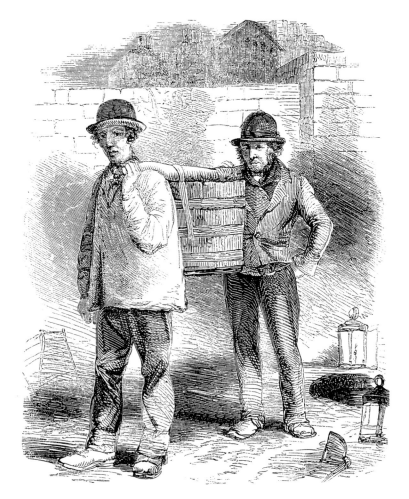

London nightmen going about their work by lantern light. They are seen carrying away the sewage, which has been scooped out of the open cesspit using long-handled scoops. From Mayhew's *London Labour and the London Poor*, 1861.

fill the tub, using a ladder to descend into the pit when the level dropped. The tub which could weigh as much as a hundredweight when it was full, was hoisted up by the 'ropeman'. Two 'tubmen' then raised the tub on a long pole and carried it on their shoulders to a covered cart where it was emptied. Very often the tub had to be carried through the house, 'to the excessive annoyance of the inmates', observed Mayhew. The work was hard and the men tough. Beer, bread and cheese were occasionally provided by the household: some gangs would drink a bottle of gin between them. Even though it was a frosty night, Mayhew found the smell, 'literally sickening'; the men themselves, it appears, scarcely noticed it. Finally, when the work was done the wagon or cart was drawn away, doubtless to the profound relief of the household.[32]

The carts were driven to 'nightyards' where huge piles of refuse accumulated. According to Mayhew there were about sixty such yards in London until about 1848. One at Spitalfields, he reported, contained, 'a heap of dung and refuse of every description . . . about the size of a tolerably large house'.[33] Some of those Hector Gavin encountered during his rambles around Bethnal Green consisted of several heaps of 'filth, dust, dirt and ashes mixed with decaying animal and vegetable remains and manure of all kinds'. Of another he said, 'the odour given off from this place is beyond conception disgusting – it spreads to a great distance and is complained of by all as an intolerable nuisance'.[34] The nightsoil was allowed to desiccate before being sold as manure to farmers and gardeners. Large quantities of nightsoil were transported by barge up the Grand Union Canal to farms in Hertfordshire and around the coast to Southampton Water where it was sold to farmers in Hampshire.[35] However, the London nightyards were suppressed after the passing of sanitary measures in September 1848.[36] There were several 'scavengers yards' in

Handbill for G. Hardy, chimney sweeper and nightman, Black Horse Yard, Rathbone Place, Oxford Street, London, *c.* 1800. At the bottom of the bill two nightmen are seen carrying a filled tub slung over a pole to the covered cart. (*Bristol City Museum and Art Gallery*)

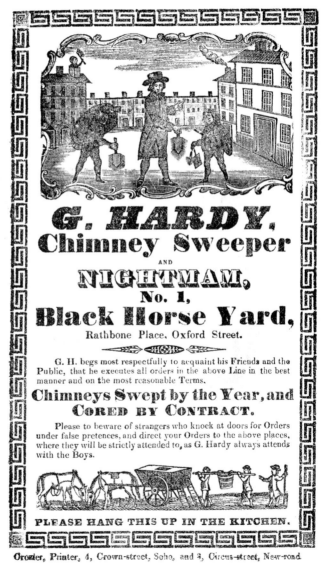

Bristol in 1850. One of three in Ashton, an untidy industrial area south of the city, was close to a group of cottages. It was the subject of many complaints: cholera was reported as being bad there.[37]

In rural areas, George Wilson believed the midden system was not objectionable because the pits could be cleaned out 'without creating a nuisance'. Disposal was easier too: the nightsoil could be buried in trenches in gardens.[38] But in towns the stench from the decomposition of these 'filth accumulations' so often situated close to the houses was seriously detrimental to health.[39] The evidence collected under Edwin Chadwick's supervision for his *Report into the Sanitary Condition of the Labouring Population of Great Britain*, published in 1842, drew public attention, for the first time, to the atrocious sanitary conditions prevailing in most towns – particularly in the poorer quarters. Further evidence was published in 1844 and 1845 by the Health of Towns Commission. Chadwick was again responsible. He sent commissioners to report on conditions in fifty towns with the highest death rates. During their visit to Bristol, one of the two investigators, Sir Henry de la Beche (1796–1855), had to stand at the end of alleys in the poor and grossly overcrowded parts of the city and vomit while his colleague, Dr Lyon Playfair (1818–98), inspected overflowing privies.[40]

A survey of the sanitary state of Bethnal Green on the eastern outskirts of London by Hector Gavin, in 1848, revealed appalling conditions. In Helen's Place he found four one-room houses – mere sheds – which shared a privy. 'The cesspool is nearly full,' he wrote, 'the wood work of the privy can scarcely hold together and it is dangerous to use it. Not long ago the landlady of some houses in Armstrong-buildings fell into a cesspool and was suffocated. Such an event is extremely probable here from the dilapidated condition of the place.' Gavin found that the removal of the soil from privies in Bethnal Green was often postponed for as long as possible, partly because of the expense but also because it was such a disgusting event. The landlords of the poorer tenements rarely emptied the cesspools and privies until fever struck, only then would they take action to prevent their property acquiring a bad name and losing tenants. The poor sometimes attempted to take action themselves, burying the soil in their yards only to contaminate the well water which was often in the same yard. Elsewhere in Bethnal Green, Gavin found privies without 'regular cesspools', some located close to the house entrance: most were full and some overflowing. Many of the houses were extremely dilapidated and in an 'excessively filthy state'. Few had a supply of water or proper drainage. 'It is nearly the universal custom,' Gavin observed, 'to throw refuse water and garbage on the streets. Some privies had very small cesspools placed

'Many of the privies are wooden sheds erected over holes from which a surface hollow conducts off the surface fluid refuse to some other part of the ground.'
Hector Gavin on Bethnal Green, 1848.

above ditches so their contents would drain into them – the ditches were filled with every imaginable type of rubbish, including dead cats and dogs in various states of decay.'[41] Similar conditions prevailed in the other poor parishes of London. An inquiry into water supply and drainage in some London parishes by the Board of Health, undertaken in 1850, revealed that in the parish of St George the Martyr, Southwark, privies were present in 97.03 per cent of houses: only a little over 10 per cent had water closets.[42] Most evidence of this sort was collected by middle-class professional investigators, but in July 1849, an extraordinary letter appeared in *The Times*. It was signed by 54 residents of Church Lane and Carrier Street, part of a crowded 'rookery' in the parish of St Giles, where 2,850 people lived in 95 houses covering little more than an acre. In crude and misspelt English, the letter described the squalor they had to endure: 'We live in Mucke and filthe. We aint got no priviz, no dust bins, no drains, no water supplies and no drain or suer in the wholeplace.'[43]

> *'We live in Mucke and filthe. We aint got no priviz, no dust bins, no drains, no water supplies and no drain or suer in the whole place.'*
> Fifty-four residents of Church Lane and Carrier Street, London to *The Times*, 1849.

In the second half of the nineteenth century, the primitive privy-midden was slowly replaced in towns either by improved dry closets* or water closets. From the 1840s successive governments passed legislation directed at improving levels of cleanliness and health in the rapidly expanding towns: by 1850 roughly 50 per cent of the country's population was urban. In London, the Metropolitan Sewers Act of 1848 forbade the construction of new houses without a water closet or privy and created a body, the Metropolitan Commission of Sewers, which began the work of removing cesspools: within about 6 years, 30,000 had been abolished.[44] The first Public Health Act of 1848 established a General Board of Health at national level and enabled local boards of health to be created in districts where the death rate exceeded 23 per 1,000. These local bodies tackled a wide range of sanitary issues – from improving drainage, water supply and ventilation to the problems of unregulated slaughter houses and even overcrowded graveyards. In Liverpool the corporation forbade the construction of new houses without water closets in 1860 and began the conversion from existing cesspits and privies to water closets in 1863.[45] In Bristol, the corporation created a local board of health in 1851 called the Sanitary Committee. During the 1850s and 1860s, the committee developed an integrated system of sewers and tackled a whole range of 'nuisances' making use of its powers under the Nuisances Removal Act of 1855. Proceedings were taken against the owners of filthy privies. A typical example was an order of October

---

*   See chapter three.

1857 to Frederick Bull, a resident of Bedminster, a rapidly growing working-class suburb south of the City Docks, requiring him to remove an offensive privy and build two new closets with connections to the new sewer. By 1869, *The Times* reported that Bristol had been transformed 'from nearly the most unhealthy to be nearly the most healthy town in Great Britain'.[46] The Public Health Act of 1875 further strengthened the hand of local authorities to act against nuisances and the inadequate provision of closets or privies.[47] The worst horrors of foul and noisome privies shared by several households were finally eradicated.

Gradually, from the 1850s, the connection between cholera and other infectious diseases and polluted water was established. But it took time, so firmly entrenched was the miasma theory. In 1849 Dr John Snow (1813–58), a pioneering anaesthetist, had suggested that water polluted by sewage might be the means by which cholera was transmitted. During the cholera epidemic of 1854, he observed a high incidence of the disease among residents in Soho, London, who drew their water from a public pump in Broad Street. He then discovered a sewer ran by. The local parish officials promptly removed the handle of the pump but the miasma theory continued to influence leading sanitarians such as Chadwick who remained convinced that bad air caused disease. Attitudes only began to change following another outbreak of cholera in the capital in 1866. The deaths were largely confined to several East End parishes supplied with water by the East London Water Co. The water was found to contain sewage and the value of Snow's pioneering work was belatedly recognised. Finally, in 1883, Robert Koch (1843–1910), a German bacteriologist, identified the cholera bacillus in India and established that it was conveyed in polluted water contaminated by the faeces of sufferers of the disease.

At last, the real danger to health presented by leaking privy-middens and cesspools was exposed. Privies were not outlawed, but fundamental changes to their design and construction and the way they were managed were introduced. Privies would be safer if they were made watertight, so guidelines for the siting and construction of privies were drawn up by the Local Government Board and published as model by-laws in about 1890. They were to be located at least 6 ft from a house and a minimum of 60 ft from a well, spring or stream. Floors were to be at least 6 in above the surrounding ground and made with flagstones or tiles or some other non-absorbent material. If the receptacle for filth was fixed it had to be provided with 'the means for the effectual application of ashes, dust or dry refuse to any filth deposited in such receptacle'.[48] Many local authorities adopted these recommendations and passed by-laws to

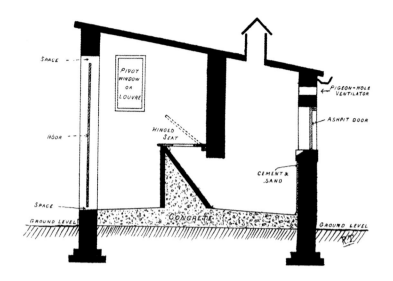

SPACE

PIVOT
WINDOW
OR
LOUVRE

PIGEON-HOLE
VENTILATOR

ASHPIT DOOR

HINGED
SEAT

FLOOR

CEMENT &
SAND

SPACE

GROUND LEVEL

CONCRETE

GROUND LEVEL

An improved privy-midden designed according to the model by-laws drawn up by the Local Government Board in about 1890. The privy was to be built a minimum of 6 ft from a dwelling house in towns, with the assumption that the distance would be greater in the countryside. The privy is well ventilated and has a non-porous floor not less than 6 in above the surrounding ground. A hatch for depositing ash or earth is provided at the back and access (not shown) for cleaning out the waste was also usually provided near ground level.

ensure they were followed.[49] The ancient privy-midden was, in effect, transformed from a wet into a dry privy, a considerably safer and more sanitary device. The responsibility for providing the waste receptacles and their regular emptying was undertaken by the local authority. By the end of the nineteenth century the old type of privy-midden was a thing of the past in towns and cities.

In many rural districts, however, the old privy-midden lasted well into the twentieth century and many of them fell far short of the standards set by the model by-laws. Writing in 1915, William Savage, the medical officer of health for Somerset said, 'where there are no drains . . . the old fashioned and utterly detestable privy-midden is still the commonest form of receptacle for excreta. These are steadily, but scarcely rapidly, being replaced either by water closets or by bucket closets.'[50] Converted to dry closets using buckets, ash or earth, many old privies continued in use for several more decades until they also became objects of curiosity to a society accustomed to using water closets. But the paradox was that of the two, the water closet was the older device. The pail closet may have appeared primitive but it was, in reality, a relatively modern device, introduced in the 1860s. The history of the water closet, however, can be traced with little difficulty to the sixteenth century.

CHAPTER TWO

Down the Pan

the first water closets

Simple privies – middens or bogs – may have varied in detail and gone by many names, but most had one unattractive feature in common: the seat and the human waste remained close companions for quite some time. Until the pit or space below the seat was emptied, human sewage piled up causing an abominable stench, frequently contaminating nearby sources of water and spreading the risk of disease. Some privies were situated over running water so that the waste was carried away downstream. The water closet worked on a similar principle, except, instead of a continuous flow of water, a sudden flush was released to remove the waste via a drain to somewhere else.

Sir John Harington (1561–1612), attributed to Hieronimo Custodis, fl.1589. (*National Portrait Gallery*)

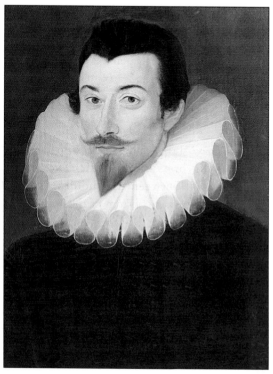

Mention water closets and the name Thomas Crapper soon crops up. In the popular mind he is often seen as the brains behind the invention of this essential component of the civilised world. With a name that could have come straight out of a novel by Charles Dickens, this ingenious Victorian plumber solved one of man's oldest problems while obligingly giving his name to the slang verb to 'crap' and the less than flattering adjective 'crap'. The idea is, of course, pure fiction – or even absolute crap – although the man did exist and he was a Victorian sanitary engineer with works in Chelsea, London. But long before his business was established in 1861, water closets were being manufactured, installed and flushed; patents were being taken out for improvements to their working and the patentees arguing in court over infringements to their patent rights. And intriguingly, the use of the word 'crap' to signify the physical act that made water closets so essential also predates Thomas Crapper's arrival in the world of sanitary science.[1]

Some 300 years earlier, a water closet designed to impress royalty made a well-publicised debut. It was designed by Sir John Harington (1561–1612), a godson of Elizabeth I. He installed it at his house at Kelston, near Bath, in readiness for a visit of the queen in 1592 when he was serving as High Sheriff of Somerset: it must have met with royal approval as one was subsequently installed in Richmond Palace. Neither device survives and Harington's house at Kelston was later demolished, but his fame as an early inventor of the water closet rests on his book, *A New Discourse on a Stale Subject: Called the Metamorphosis of Ajax*, published in 1596. Ajax was a pun on 'jakes', a slang word for privy or closet used widely at the time. In this light-hearted book Harington gave instructions on how to transform 'your worst privy' so that it was, 'as sweet as your best chamber', and all for 30*s* 8*d*.

The water closet consisted of a straight-sided oval 'stool pot' with a base that sloped to one side where a brass 'sluice or washer' was fitted. This could be opened or closed by turning a vertical iron rod which had a turning key behind the seat. The seat itself was the usual round hole cut out of a plank but had a small V at the front – 'a peak devant for elbow room', Harington explained. The device was flushed by opening a 'cock or washer' in a lead pipe which brought water from an overhead cistern to just below the seat. Harington recommended lining the pot with pitch, rosin and wax to prevent it from being tainted with urine. He also emphasised that the closet should be carefully sealed with plaster so the only connection with the 'vault' (i.e. cesspit) was through the brass sluice which would remain closed between use, holding six inches of water in the bottom of the pot. 'If water be clean,' wrote Harington, 'the oftener it is used and opened the sweeter', although he added that if water was scarce, a daily flush would be sufficient, 'though twenty persons should use it'.

Sir John Harington wanted his invention to bring him fame: 'I was the willinger to wryte . . . because I thought this would give me some occasion to have me thought

'If water be clean the oftener it is used and opened the sweeter.'
Sir John Harington, 1596.

Harington's improved 'jakes' of 1596 showing the water cistern (A), the seat (D) and the stool pot (H). The turning key (g) is seen beside the seat hole which has a V cut out at the front for 'elbow room'.

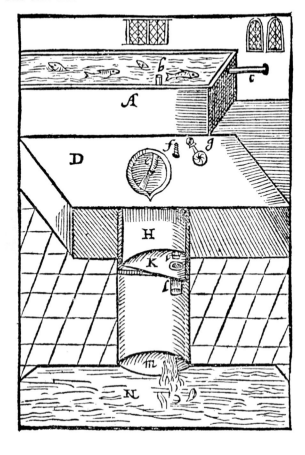

of and talked of.' But his fame was clearly limited and the idea
appears to have died with him in 1612. The first patent for a water
closet was not taken out until 1775, even though the system of
granting royal patents had started only five years after Harington's
death. Thus his closet remains something of a 'one-off' in the history
of sanitaryware – a late Elizabethan novelty – which had little or no
bearing on future developments. As it was, the impact of his
invention was bound to be restricted. Being a godson of the queen, he
was part of a small social and cultural elite. Few people would have
had access to his book – let alone be able to read it – and doubtless,
fewer still would have been prepared to spend 30s 8d on one of the
less talked of parts of the home. It is also very likely that Harington's
'metamorphosis' of the privy was not quite the original piece of
thought that he would have us believe. Although the evidence is
imprecise it appears very likely that attempts to flush closets with
water had been tried before.

But the idea may not have died altogether. Fragmentary evidence
survives to suggest that water closets may have enjoyed limited use
throughout the seventeenth century. The antiquarian John Aubrey,
writing in 1673, described a water closet he had seen at the home of
Sir Francis Carew at Bedington, Surrey: 'Here I saw a pretty machine
to cleanse an House of Office viz., by a small stream no bigger than
one's finger which ran into an engine made like a bit of a fire shovel
which hung upon its centre of gravity, so that when it was full a
considerable quantity of water fell down with some force and washed
away the filth.'[2] A similar self-acting tipping action featured in the
tumbler or tipper closets of the late nineteenth century. In 1687,
water closets with a flush were fitted in the stool room at St James's
Palace by Peter Thomson, the 'engine maker'[3] and between 1691 and
1694, at least ten were installed at Chatsworth, the seat of the Duke
of Devonshire in Derbyshire.[4] In the first half of the eighteenth
century, the idea of adding water to the closet was slowly established.
When Alexander Cummings (c. 1732–1814), a London horologist,
took out the first patent for a water closet in 1775, he made no
attempt to claim their invention; instead, his patent featured a 'water
closet upon a new construction'. Clearly, Cummings was not
introducing water closets to the world, merely an improved model.

So, how far had the adoption of water closets progressed before
Cumming's patent? Celia Fiennes (1662–1741) visited Chatsworth in
1697. She was impressed by the waterworks in the gardens and the
bath with its hot and cold water, but does not mention the water
closets which had been installed just a few years earlier. However, in
1712, on visiting Windsor, she came across a water closet in the
dressing room of Prince George at Burfield Lodge. The prince,

consort to Queen Anne, had died four years earlier, but Celia Fiennes saw a closet, 'with a seate of easement of marble with sluces of water to wash all down'.[5] In 1728, the Duke of Chandos employed John Wood to build a fashionable lodging house in Bath which was to be fully equipped with water closets and they are listed in an inventory of 1733 of the duke's own house in St James's Square, London.[6] The same year, a water closet was recorded at Lord Chesterfield's house at 45 Grosvenor Square, London.[7]

Still largely restricted to aristocratic circles, it may have been around this time that the idea found its way to France. Jacques François Blondel (d. 1774), a French professor of architecture, included designs for a *'lieux à soupage'* – a place with a valve – in an architectural work of 1737/8. According to Blondel, these devices had 'for some years come to be much used in France in houses of consequence'. They were also known in France as *'lieux à l'Anglaise'* and were believed to have been invented in England, but 'several people from that country', he added, 'tell me that they have not heard of their being used in London'.[8] Back in London, published works which might have included reference to closets supplied with water are, at best, vague. *The London Art of Building*, published in 1734, states, 'that convenient cisterns be well placed, plentifully to furnish every office with water', but there are no further details. In 1747, R. Campbell, author of *The London Tradesman* said the plumber 'makes pipes to convey water into our kitchens and office houses'.[9] Again, there is no specific mention of water closets. The French word *'lieux'* for water closet was to become the English word, 'loo', but it was to be a while yet before the device and the name became commoner than 'privy' or 'bog'.

After the 1750s, the use of water closets among the better-off appears to have become more general. In the early 1760s they were fitted into two new houses designed by Robert and John Adam: Osterly House and Syon House. In about 1879, S. Stevens Hellyer, a leading sanitary engineer and reformer, came across two water closets at Osterley House which may have been installed when the house was first built in 1761. They consisted of a marble pan with a plug waste operated by lifting a vertical rod as in Harington's closet. The pan had an overflow and a service pipe delivering clean flush water from an overhead cistern. 'A niche in a fair sized room,' wrote Hellyer in 1892, 'was formed to receive the marble closet pan, and a door, shutting up close to the seat, hid the whole arrangement from sight.' As a practical sanitary engineer, Hellyer noted also that the lead soil pipe which connected the plug waste with the drain was not ventilated. Water closet technology, therefore, had not progressed beyond Harington's 'Ajax' of 1592.

Alexander Cummings (c. 1732–1814)

LEXANDER CUMMINGS is believed to have been born in Edinburgh in about 1732. In the second half of the eighteenth century he was a leading London clock and watchmaker and was elected an honorary freeman of the Clockmaker's Company in 1781. The Clockmaker's Library has a folio volume containing memoranda, descriptions, observations and correspondence collected by Cummings between 1766 and 1812. This provides some idea of the wide range of his interests in mechanical and scientific matters including barometrics, hydraulics and centrifugal force. He is credited with the invention of a clock escapement and made a barometric recording clock for George III. In 1766 he wrote *The Elements of Clock and Watch Work* and also assisted the Board of Longitude in laying down the conditions for the testing of Harrison's fourth marine chronometer. At the time of his 1775 patent for water closets he was working at 'The Dial and Three Crowns' in New Bond Street. He died at Pentonville in 1814.

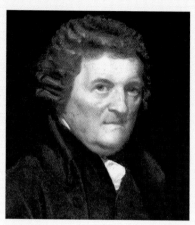

Alexander Cummings. (*The Worshipful Company of Clockmakers*)

Fourteen years after the initial building of Osterly House, Alexander Cummings, (*c.* 1732–1814) the Bond Street watchmaker and leading horologist, was granted a royal patent for his improved water closet. Several important innovations were incorporated in his design and one in particular provided further illustration that water closets must have been familiar in London by this time. 'The stink trap hitherto used for water closets,' wrote Cummings in his patent specification, 'is too well known to require a description here.' Without a seal sewer gases could enter a room through the closet, so it was essential that a water-sealed trap was fitted below the device. This had been imperfectly understood by Wood in Bath in 1728, but the use of traps must have spread by the 1770s, and the type which Cummings was all too aware of was almost certainly the so-called D trap. This trap was widely used as it was a straightforward matter for a plumber to make one from pieces of sheet lead soldered together. While it cut off the foul smells from the drain, the D trap unfortunately generated its own, as the water it contained was not completely replaced by the flush water. It was not, in other words, self-cleaning. As Cummings pointed out, 'it becomes in itself a magazine of foetid matter, which emits an offensive smell every time that it is disturbed by using the water closet'. Instead, he specified a trap which was 'recurved' about 12 or 18 in below the pan so that it held sufficient 'stagnated water' to cut off all smells from below and which, 'is totally emptied and succeeded by fresh [water] every time the pan or bason is emptied'.

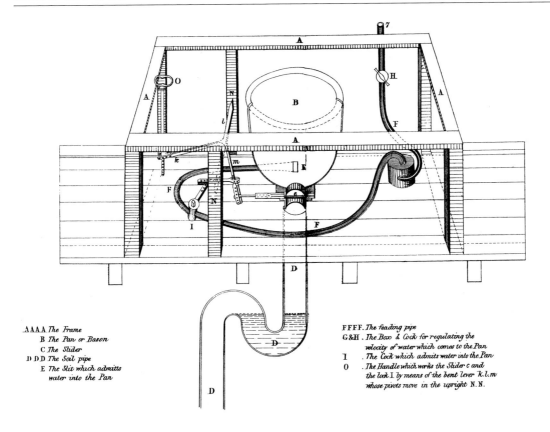

AAAA *The Frame*
  B *The Pan or Bason*
  C *The Slider*
D DD *The Soil pipe*
  E *The Slit which admitts*
    water into the Pan

FFFF. *The feeding pipe*
G &H . *The Box & Cock for regulating the*
    velocity of water which comes to the Pan
  I   . *The Cock which admits water into the Pan*
  O   . *The Handle which works the Slider c and*
    the cock I by means of the bent lever k.l.m
    whose pivots move in the upright N.N.

The introduction of the water-sealed trap – popularly known as the U bend – was, in itself, an important development, but Cummings also introduced other improvements to the water closet. The seal to the soil pipe was further protected by an outlet valve at the bottom of the pan. This was operated by a handle and angled lever: when the handle was pulled up the lever drew the valve or 'slider' to one side. Simultaneously, the cock or inlet valve which released the flush water was opened by a lever working off the main one controlling the sliding valve. This simultaneous action of the inlet and outlet valves was to remain a basic feature of all valve closets until their demise in the early twentieth century. Cummings made the pan circular with the deepest part under the middle of the seat to ensure that the 'soil' – to use the patentee's own word – would be deposited near the outlet and submerged in the water held in the bottom of the pan by a sliding valve. The flush water, instead of pouring into the pan from a pipe or spout just below the seat, entered through a rectangular slit placed just 4 or 5 in above the outlet. As Cummings explained, 'The water entering the pan or bason through this slit with rapidity is circulated and accumulated within it, so as to wash or cleanse it.'[10]

Cummings's water closet from his patent specification of 1775. The sliding valve can be seen at the bottom of the pan connected to the closet handle by an angled lever.

Cummings's water closet represented a major advance in their design, and yet its shortcomings have tended to overshadow his achievement. The main problem was the sliding valve: when it was opened, this vital component was not exposed to the cleansing action of the flush and when it returned to the shut position it remained soiled from the previous use. Over time, the valve acquired a coating of encrusted dirt; it was also prone to rust and so became increasingly difficult to move. This defect came to the attention of a young tradesman from Yorkshire, Joseph Bramah (1748–1815), who had moved to London to find work in 1773. Working as a joiner and cabinet maker for a Mr Allen, who, apparently had made his own modifications to Cummings's design, Bramah became acquainted with water closets, fitting the wooden enclosures and seats.[11] In May 1778, describing himself as a cabinet maker of Cross Court, Carnaby Market, he took out a patent for a water closet with two valves, 'so situated and constructed as totally to prevent the great inconveniences complained of in every sort of water closets heretofore made use of'.[12] Bramah replaced Cummings's 'slider' with a flap valve: this dropped down when the handle was pulled so that it was, in his own words, 'thoroughly washed every time the contents of the basin are discharged'. Bramah also moved the inlet valve from its customary position at the end of the feed pipe, near the closet bowl or pan, to high up in the cistern. He had obviously encountered many instances of the water in the feed pipe and the inlet valve freezing in cold weather. Perhaps the problem had been particularly acute during the winter of 1776 when Parson Woodforde encountered snow drifts in Oxford and in Selbourne, Hampshire, Gilbert White wrote of fierce frosts which froze the contents of chamber pots under beds.[13] With Bramah's modification there was now less likelihood of the feed pipe or valve freezing. The feed pipe was now below the valve and so was drained of water after every use. Bramah also placed the valve mechanism above the water level in the cistern so it could not be frozen in ice.

Bramah had devised an extremely effective water closet. The basin contained a good depth of water in which solids were completely submerged and liquids diluted; it had a large exposed surface of water reducing to a minimum the possibility of fouling the basin and practically silent action. His cranking arrangement, which operated the two valves, was also more effective than Cummings's design. The main lever, one end of which was raised by pulling the flushing handle, was held against a wooden board by a spring. This ensured that when the handle was released it sprung back into position and also that the flap valve was held tight against the bottom of the pan. The mechanism included a shorter lever working

'Fierce frost: ice under people's beds & cutting winds.'
Gilbert White,
28 January 1776.

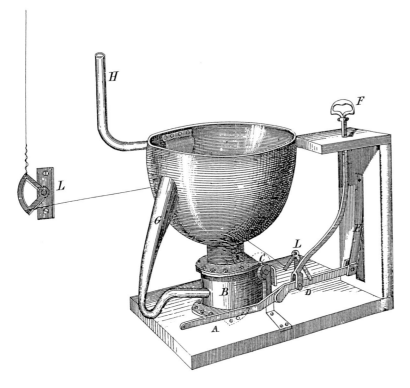

Bramah's valve closet from his patent specification of 1778. Flush water entered the closet from the pipe (H), behind a fan riveted to the pan. The waste left through the lead valve box (B). The diagram shows the closet handle (F), connected to the main lever (D), which was sprung against the vertical board and connected to a small crank (C), which operated the outlet valve. The pipe (G) is the overflow and is bent to contain a water seal from the valve box. Part of the system of wires and cranks operating the inlet valve in the cistern is seen on the left.

off the main lever so the water supply valve operated simultaneously. By the early nineteenth century, water closets controlled by a sprung lever like Bramah's were called 'spring valve closets'.

In place of a spring, many nineteenth-century Bramah-type closets used cast-iron counterweights attached to the end of the two levers: these also ensured the discharge valve snapped shut in a businesslike way. Bramah's outlet valve rotated – or flapped – within an iron valve box on which the pan or basin rested. The valve box was provided with its own ventilation and was also connected to an overflow pipe from the pan above: this overflow was made with a reverse curve to create a water-seal trap to prevent bad air from escaping from the apparatus. A short distance below the valve box was another seal – a water-seal trap – which provided a second barrier between the closet pan and the soil pipe. Bramah said nothing of this in his patent, and illustrations of valve closets as late as the 1850s suggest that they were usually fitted with the inefficient D trap. The trap was usually located under the floorboards and was, therefore, virtually impossible to get at for maintenance or cleaning, but the cranking mechanism, valve box and pan were enclosed in a wooden cabinet, usually of mahogany. The top contained the seat with its round hole above the pan and a smaller one at the side fitted with the cup and pull handle.

Joseph Bramah (1749–1814)

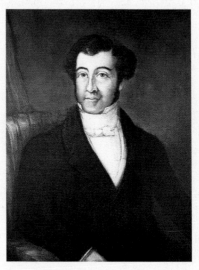

OSEPH BRAMAH was the son of a farmer from Stainborough, near Barnsley, Yorkshire. He served an apprenticeship with the village carpenter, but in 1773 decided to seek work in London. He made the journey on foot and secured work as a journeyman cabinet maker working for a Mr Allen of Cross Court, Carnaby Market. While recovering from a serious fall at work he turned his attention to improving on Cunmmings' valve closet, and in 1778 patented his own improved design – only the third to be taken out for a water closet. This was his first patent and he soon set up business on his own as a cabinet maker in the less than salubrious Denmark Street in the parish of St Giles. Bramah's valve closets were a commercial success. He could probably have established fame and success on this invention alone, but this remarkably talented and inventive man went on to take out another seventeen patents covering improvements to water cocks, locks, fire engines, carriage brakes and suspension, printing presses and even fountain pens. He also invented the hydraulic press, without which many of the great engineering feats of the nineteenth century would have been impossible.

Joseph Bramah. (*Institution of Mechanical Engineers*)

In 1783 he was elected a member of the Society of Arts, which brought him into contact with some of the leading engineers and manufacturers of the time. The following year he took out a patent for an entirely new type of lock that contained levers that could not be picked by the average picklock. Until the first patent by Chubb in 1818, Bramah had a virtual monopoly on high-class locks. In 1784 he also moved to more fashionable premises at the west end of Piccadilly. By 1785, when he took out a patent for a hydrostatical machine, he was describing himself as an engineer, and subsequently established works at Pimlico which included a foundry, machine or engineering shop, a pattern shop and a model or research room. He married Mary Lawton from near his family home in 1785 and had five children, three of whom adopted engineering as their career. The oldest, Timothy, had joined the family firm by 1813 when the name of the company changed from Bramah and Co. to Bramah and Sons, but in December 1814 Joseph Bramah died and was buried in Paddington churchyard. The firm continued in business until about 1890, by which time none of the family was involved.

Joseph Bramah was one of those rare individuals who combined a practical and inventive mind with business acumen. Having somehow raised the £120 required to take out a patent he soon established his own premises in the heart of the fashionable West End at 124 Piccadilly. Bramah's closets were not cheap: in the 1780s and 1790s, his 'patent apparatus' cost 8 guineas but the total cost, including the cistern, valve and pipe-work came to over £11. Nevertheless, this was the first water closet to enjoy major commercial success. He soon attracted imitators, including a certain Hardcastle, who he took to court in 1789 for infringing his patent; witnesses vouched for the superiority of Bramah's device over previous ones and he won his case.[14] He attracted custom nationwide. In 1787, he supplied one of his 'patent apparatus' to Soho House in Birmingham, the home of Mathew Boulton, the

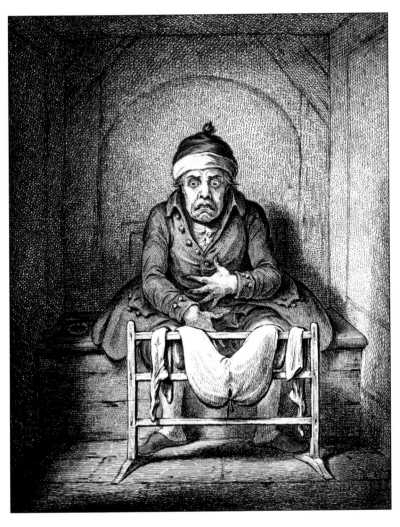

'Brisk Cathartic'. Early water closets were contained in a wooden enclosure and superficially resembled the primitive privy; however, the pull handle in the seat seen to the right of the user indicates that this is a water closet. Attributed to Gillray, published by W. Humphrey, London, 28 January 1804. (*British Museum*)

leading industrialist.[15] Six years later, he was supplying another four to the country seat of Thomas Anson at Shugborough Hall, near Lichfield, Staffordshire.[16] The owners of large country houses often equipped and furnished their homes from leading London suppliers, and situated in Piccadilly, Bramah was well placed to pick up provincial business. By 1797 he claimed to have sold 6,000 of his closets. Bramah's inventiveness and business flair quickly moved on to other areas – he made important improvements to locks and pioneered the hydraulic press – but his success as a manufacturer of water closets was secured. In the nineteenth century the Bramah became the accepted water closet among the well-to-do and his name a byword for the valve closet.

Bramah was not alone, however, in developing the water closet, and by 1800, seven patents had been taken out for water closets. In 1777, Lemuel Prosser, a London plumber, patented a closet with a

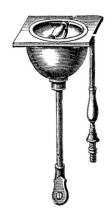

A closet handle for a pan closet, 1889. The handle, made of cut glass, ebony or china, was set in a brass cup recessed into the seat.

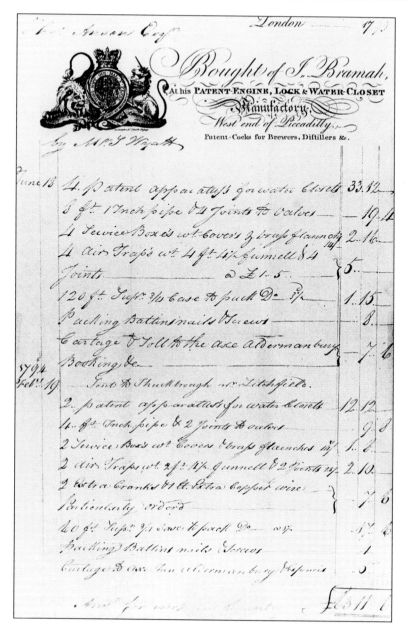

A bill for six water closets or 'patent apparatus' from Joseph Bramah, water-closet manufacturer, Piccadilly, London, to Thomas Anson of Shugborough Hall, Staffordshire, 1793/4. The bill also lists the service boxes supplying the flush water, traps, valves and pipes. (*Staffordshire Record Office*)

plug set in a vertical tube. However, he submitted virtually no explanation in his patent other than vague and simple diagrams which suggest foul water would have circulated freely from the pan to the tube.[17] Fortunately for posterity, the name 'Prosser' never became synonymous with the water closet. In 1796, William Law, a London iron founder, took out a patent for a self-acting closet where the flush was released upon the user rising from the seat. His patent featured a type of closet which was to become the chief rival of the Bramah closet in the nineteenth century.[18] This was the pan closet, so named –

not after the upper bowl or pan – but after a metal pan that took the place of the outlet valve, holding water in the upper bowl and creating a seal. When the flushing handle was pulled the pan tipped the waste downwards. The pan closet was clearly in use before the mid-1790s. Law did not lay claim to its invention in his patent – just his self-acting device – and an example from Hampton Court, which is believed to date from about 1780, survives intact, albeit somewhat battered and incomplete in the Science Museum, London.[19]

This sudden flurry of patents for water closets from the 1770s occurred at a time when material standards of living were rapidly improving. In short, people were becoming more civilised: contemporaries noticed the difference between England in the 1740s and the 1780s. Expectations of comfort in the home – at least, for the better-off – were rising and they were met by new manufacturers producing a wider range of consumer goods – from fine earthenware and carpets to cast-iron grates and ovens. Between about 1750 and 1800, several important developments took place in domestic furnishings and equipment: fireplaces and cooking facilities were improved; from the 1780s, the first good-quality oil lamps were manufactured in Birmingham, and the following decade the practicality of using gas for lighting was established. The improvement in the design of the water closet, therefore, was no isolated phenomenon but part of a wider consumer revolution which transformed levels of comfort, at least for the upper and middle classes.

By the early 1800s, the manufacture of water closets by plumbers and brass founders was established in most large towns and cities. It coincided with the start of a boom in the building trade. The rate of house building grew steadily in the early decades of the nineteenth

'All the better class of closets in mansions built about twenty or thirty years ago will be found mostly supplied with this pattern.'
William Eassie on Bramah closets, 1872.

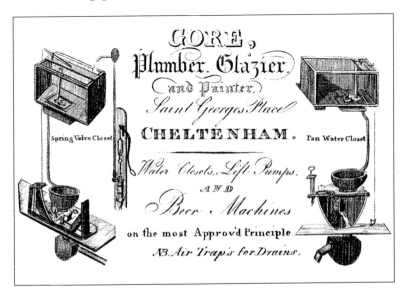

An advertisement for water closets by Gore, plumber, glazier and painter, in St George's Place, Cheltenham from J.K. Griffith, *A General Cheltenham Guide*, 1818. The two water closets are shown complete with overhead cisterns and D traps. The valve closet is fitted with a sprung lever operating the mechanism and is shown with a hand pump supplying the cistern. On the right the pan closet is shown in action with the hand pull up and the rotating pan tipping the waste into the trap. (*Cheltenham Library*)

Thomas Crapper (1837–1910)

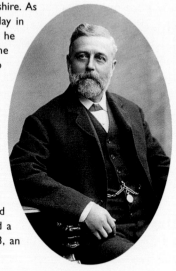

Thomas Crapper. (*Thomas Crapper and Co. Ltd*)

THOMAS CRAPPER was born in Thorne, near Doncaster, Yorkshire. As a young boy, he appears to have decided that his future lay in London, and aged only eleven walked to the capital where he found employment with a plumber in Chelsea. In 1861 he established his own business in Robert Street, and in 1866 moved to Marlborough Road where he established a manufactory including a brass works.

In spite of his fame, Crapper actually had very little to do with the development of the water closet. No major stages in its development are attributable to him, although he took out a patent for a self-rising closet seat in 1863 and another in 1902 for a trough closet fitted with water-sealed traps under each unit. His biographer, Wallace Reyburn, has emphasised his role in developing water waste preventing cisterns, but he was not responsible for any major improvements in these either. By the time he took out a patent for automatic flushing cisterns in 1891, 'pull and let go' syphonic cisterns were already well established. He also patented a disconnecting trap for drains, a seat-action automatic flush and, in 1903, an improved type of stair tread.

Thomas Crapper's place in the history of sanitary equipment, therefore, is not that of a pioneer, but rather as a representative of the many Victorian sanitaryware manufacturers who profited from efforts to improve standards of public health and domestic sanitation from the 1840s. Like many sanitary engineers, Crapper's technical skills were based in metal working – in his case, plumbing and brass founding – and not potting. Crapper produced a wide range of sanitary fittings including domestic ware – such as the attractive ceramic pedestal closet, the 'Marlboro', introduced in 1887 – and drain components. Cast-iron man-holes bearing his name are widely found: there are three in Westminster Abbey. In 1886 he was granted a royal warrant after installing new sanitary fittings at Sandringham House, the home of the Prince of Wales.

In 1907 the firm moved to 120 Kings Road, Chelsea and Thomas sold the business to his old partner, Robert Wareham and his nephew, George Crapper. He was remembered as a genial man of average height with a grey beard similar to that of George V. He died in 1910 and is buried in Elmers End Cemetery, south-east London. The firm continued to trade independently until 1966 when it was taken over by John Bolding and Co. who went bankrupt in 1969. Crapper and Co. was sold to another firm and lay dormant until acquired by Simon Kirby in 1999. Now back in business at Alscott Park, Stratford-on-Avon, Thomas Crapper and Co.'s range includes a water closet, the 'Venerable', cast-iron cisterns and lavatory basins based on items produced by the company in the late nineteenth century.

century reaching a peak in the 1820s and only falling off in the 1840s and 1850s. Late Georgian terraces, squares, crescents and detached villas were developed in new middle-class suburbs such as Highbury and Islington in London and Clifton in Bristol. Fashionable brick or stuccoed houses were built in spa towns like Cheltenham, Tunbridge Wells and Leamington and in seaside towns such as Brighton and Scarborough.[20] These late Georgian town houses were probably the first major category of housing to have water closets as more or less a standard fitting. They occasionally appear in contemporary advertisements of houses for sale or to let: for example, in 1833, the auction particulars for Walcot House, 'a most comfortable and gentlemanly residence' on the London Road, Bath, included two 'patent' water closets.[21] By 1821, when James Jennings compiled his *Family Cyclopaedia*, the water closet was sufficiently well known for him to describe it as 'a useful contrivance, the purpose of which requires no explanation'.[22] Looking back in 1861, Henry Mayhew reckoned Bramah's valve closet had been 'brought into general use' around the late 1820s,[23] and in 1891 S. Stevens Hellyer gave a similar date for the adoption of the pan closet.[24] A Board of Health investigation in London in 1850 found that in the prosperous parish of St James, 65.86 per cent of houses had a water closet and 45.99 per cent in the less fashionable parish of St Anne's, Soho.[25] And having a water closet, as Mayhew observed, made quite a difference: 'The houses of the rich owing to the refuse being drained away from the premises, improved both in wholesomeness and agreeableness.'

Improvements continued to be made to both valve and pan closets. It was not long before earthenware replaced cast iron for the basins. Earthenware was easier to keep clean, did not rust and was more attractive. By 1802 Wedgwood were making earthenware water closet basins for several water-closet manufacturers, including Joseph Bramah. The most expensive closets were supplied with basins decorated with underglaze transfer decoration: Italian or classical landscapes in blue and white were particular favourites. Another important feature of pans was the fan or flushing spreader, a semi-circular piece of copper riveted to the pan in front of the inlet which spread the water into a wide fan inside the bowl. Bramah showed one in his patent of 1778. More effective still was to curl over the rim of the bowl to make a flushing rim so the incoming flush water was carried around the whole interior. The first patent for a flushing rim was taken out in 1855 by Edmund Sharpe, a sanitaryware potter in Swadlincote, south Derbyshire, but it is clear they were being made before this. Sharpe's patent describes an improved flushing rim, not the original concept.[26] Regulating the supply of flush water increasingly became a preoccupation of sanitary engineers to ensure an adequate quantity of flush water entered the pan while preventing undue waste. From the 1850s most valve and pan closets were fitted with a copper or brass cylinder and piston connected to the lever controlling the inlet valve. First patented by Frederick George Underhay, a London sanitary engineer, in 1852, these regulators delayed the closing of the inlet valve so that clean water continued to flow into the bowl after the handle had been released.*

'I consider the pan closet objectionable. The "container" is usually a reservoir coated with filth hidden by the pan holding the water in the basin.' T. Mellard Reade, Liverpool, 1884.

---

* See chapter eight.

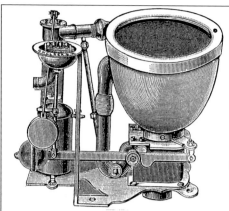
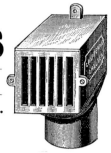

THOMAS CRAPPER & CO.'S
SANITARY
APPLIANCES

Catalogue on application.

THOMAS CRAPPER & CO.
[1]   Marlboro' Works,
CHELSEA, LONDON, S.W

Valve closets continued to be made throughout the nineteenth century. There was really very little wrong with them although the outlet valve – like all valves – was sometimes a source of trouble: it was important that they were correctly seated against the opening or water would be lost, draining the pan or basin of its water seal. Worn valves, therefore, occasionally had to be replaced. By the 1850s, valves were being made with a surface of india-rubber to provide a better seal. Valve closets did not react well to hurried or casual use: the flushing handle had to be pulled up with a precise and complete action to ensure the outlet valve opened to its full extent or blockages could occur. The cranking mechanism was another source of weakness, as it was liable to breakdown. But it is a testimony to the basic effectiveness of the design that they survived the introduction of the all-ceramic pedestal water closet in the 1880s and continued in limited production until the 1930s.

Pan closets also had their supporters. In 1857 J.H. Walsh declared, 'nothing . . . in my opinion comes up to the construction which has been so many years in use and is called the pan closet'.[27] The pan closet did have advantages over the valve closet: it was much cheaper, it was robust and able to withstand rough usage. The pan was a sure way of maintaining the water seal in the bottom of the basin: there was no possibility of water seeping away as there was through a faulty valve. There must have been occasions when the sturdy reliability of a pan closet was contrasted favourably with the more expensive but temperamental valve closet, but gradually the pan closet was exposed as a filthy, insanitary device. Edwin Chadwick, the leading sanitary reformer, was an early critic of the pan closet: by the 1870s his lone voice had turned to a chorus of condemnation from leading sanitary engineers.[28]

First, there was William Eassie, an engineer and prominent sanitarian, who in 1872 wrote, 'I cannot recommend these pan

A trade advertisement for Thomas Crapper and Co., showing a valve closet and drain air inlet, 1889. The company continued to make valve closets until the 1930s. (*Thomas Crapper and Co. Ltd*)

closets', and then in 1877, the drainage specialist, J. Bailey Denton, warned that, 'pan closets should be looked upon with suspicion'.[29] At first glance, however, the pan closet looked every bit as respectable as its more expensive counterpart, the valve closet: there was the same mahogany cabinet and seat, a smart-looking flushing handle and an earthenware bowl, perhaps in blue and white. All the features of the pan closet which made it notoriously insanitary were out of sight. The essential component was the pan which was held by a counterweight up against the outer edge of the bottom of the basin: all that could be seen of this was the inner surface of the base. What could not be seen was that when the flushing handle was pulled this pan tipped the foul water and excrement into a larger lower vessel of iron which was called the receiver. This was the equivalent of the valve box of the Bramah closet, but to accommodate the tipping action of the pan it was considerably larger. From there the waste matter passed to the soil pipe via a large D-shaped trap placed under the floor. The metal parts of the pan closet were impossible to clean: the receiver and pan accumulated filth because, in Hellyer's words, 'no frictional flush can be sent over the interior surfaces of the pan closet'. Hellyer reckoned that, on average, the metal pan of an old pan closet accumulated 2lb of dried excrement; the only way it could be effectively cleaned was to detach it and burn off the dirt in the kitchen fire.[30] The receiver, however, was impossible to get at, short of stripping down the device, so that in plumbers' parlance it could be 'taken up to be sweetened'.

The defects of the pan closet were compounded by the equally insanitary D trap. This was too large was to be emptied by the flush and retained foul water; so instead of acting as a barrier to foul air in the drain, it passed it to the room. Being under the floor, the trap was impossible to get at. 'The puffs of nasty smells', wrote Hellyer, in 1877, 'which such apparatus send up are enough to make one wish for the old privy again.' The pan closet and D trap was condemned again two years later by William Eassie, in a lecture at the Sanitary Exhibition at Croydon. 'I should, above all, like to see abolished the filthy D trap, with its furrings of foecal matter, the huge iron container with its linings of ancient ordure and the trap at the foot of the soil pipe with its excremental cesspit.'[31] Many attempts were made to improve pan closets, including reducing the size of the container, increasing the depth of the pan and lining the interior of the receiver with porcelain enamel, but the basic problem remained: the pan closet collected dirt and, moreover, it smelled. But poorly

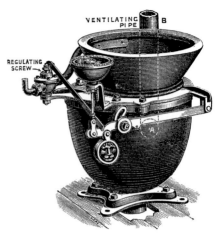

The 'Lambeth' pan closet, by Doulton and Co., 1889. The straight-sided earthenware pan sits on a cast-iron plate fixed to the top of the receiver; the cranking mechanism is also attached to this plate. The weight attached to the main lever, decorated with a lion's head, ensures the lever and pan return to the closed position when the closet handle is released. A second lever, extending as far as the regulating screw, controls the inlet valve admitting flush water behind the fan just visible in the pan.

'I should above all like to see abolished the filthy D trap with its furrings of faecal matter.'

William Eassie, 1879.

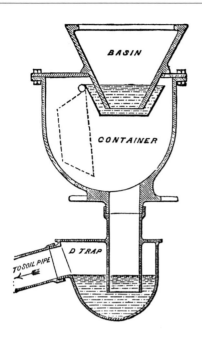 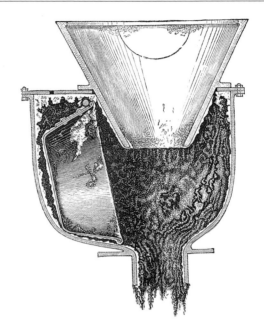

designed and complicated, water closets created a more serious problem. Early nineteenth-century water-closet technology, however imperfect, had outstripped that of sewage disposal. So, once the device was flushed and the excrement and foul water went down the pan, precisely where did it go? Before the 1860s, the answer was often, not very far . . .

In 1849, a Mr A. Cooper of Leicester wrote to the town's Highways and Sewage Committee requesting that the nearest sewer was extended towards his house for his water closet or that a drain was installed to join it. He explained, 'I am anxious that one or other should be done as a sanitary measure, for unless it be done I shall be compelled to allow some filthy and offensive water from a closet . . . to run on the surface until it reach the first grate.'[32] While the use of water closets in middle-class homes had increased dramatically over the previous twenty years, many had no connection to sewers. In 1851, Mayhew reckoned that about 50 per cent of London's houses lacked drainage to sewers; in other towns the figure was probably higher.[33] The waste from many water closets went no further than the backyard or garden of the property where it accumulated in a cesspool. And then the waste from some – like Mr Cooper's in Leicester – could even end up running down the street until it eventually found a drain. For others, the liquid sewage travelled a little further – through a brick sewer to the nearest stretch of water – where it contributed to the rapid deterioration of river water in most towns between 1800 and 1850. The coming of

Two sections of a pan closet illustrating how the closet accumulated dirt. *Left*: the tipping pan is shown closed, holding the seal of water in the earthenware basin. The inefficient D trap is below floor level and impossible to get at without removing the closet and some of the floor. *Right*: the tipping pan inclined, pouring the waste into the iron receiver where dried excrement gradually built up over the inner surfaces which could not be reached without dismantling the device.

the water closet, therefore, was something of a mixed blessing. As Henry Austin observed among the mire and dirt of Worcester in 1847, water closets 'may be said to be an evil rather than a benefit'.[34] By discharging into cesspools they tended to increase the saturation of the soil and created the same dangers to health as the privy-midden. Generating large quantities of liquid raw sewage which went nowhere in particular, the water closet, therefore, turned a private nuisance into a major public one.

Some of the cesspools which received the sewage from water closets were as crudely made as those associated with privies. In 1844, in the course of their fieldwork for the Health of Towns Commission report, Sir Henry de la Beche and Dr Lyon Playfair discovered large houses in Clifton, Bristol's wealthiest suburb, 'inhabited by persons in affluent and easy circumstances' which lacked proper sewerage. 'Ranges of handsome houses,' Sir Henry reported, 'otherwise well appointed, have nothing but a system of cesspools – often the holes from which the stones for building the chief and rough parts of the houses have been taken.'[35] The flush water of closets added considerably to the liquid bulk of the waste, and like the older bog holes and soil tanks, cesspools connected to water closets were usually made so the liquid content could seep away. In parts of London by 1840, according to Joseph Quick,

A satirical view of the disease-infested waters of the River Thames from *Punch*, 3 July 1858. Father Thames introduces his three children, Diphtheria, Scrofula, and Cholera to the Fair City of London, who, in the circumstances, looks remarkably calm. In 1851 *Punch* had referred to the Thames as the 'Great Tidal Drain'.

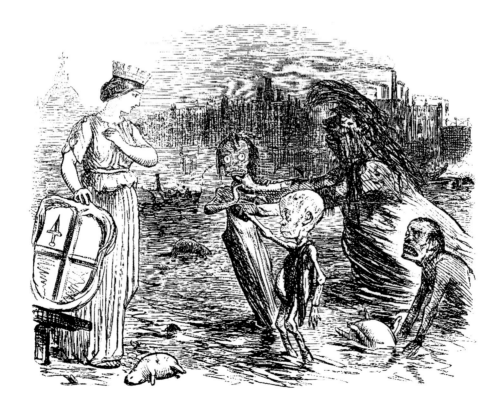

engineer to the Southwark Water Company, cesspools were being sunk as deep as the first stratum of sand so the natural drainage of their liquid contents left a smaller solid residue to be removed.[36] The release of raw, liquid sewage into the substratum of sand contaminated wells and water courses, adding to the risk of cholera and typhoid. In Bristol, Dr William Budd traced an outbreak of typhoid in Richmond Terrace – one of Clifton's fashionable terraces – to the contamination of the domestic water supply from the cesspools in the backyards.[37] It was something of a surprise for public-health investigators to discover that inadequate domestic sanitation was not confined solely to the poorer quarters of large towns. Behind splendidly furnished homes – and sometimes actually underneath them – foul-smelling and dangerous repositories of human filth represented a major threat to life.

For the new bodies created at national and local level from the 1840s to improve public health, advancing the means of disposal of water-borne sewage was as pressing an issue as removing over-crowded privy-middens and towering heaps of nightsoil. Some authorities, as in Manchester, attempted to reduce the problem by discouraging the use of water closets altogether. In common with many northern towns, Manchester, instead, turned to the development of various types of dry privies. In Birmingham, opinion was divided with water closets and dry privies both having their supporters. In the 1870s, the split appears to have followed political lines with the town's forceful Liberal mayor, Joseph Chamberlain (1836–1914), promoting the cause of clean water and effective drainage on the rates. Liverpool in contrast, was early to develop a water carriage system – possibly because of the desire to install services to aid land speculation. The Mersey also provided a convenient outlet for the sewers. Between 1847 and 1868 a mains sewer system was installed, designed by the newly appointed borough engineer, James Newlands, which expanded an earlier system designed by John Rennie (1761–1821). The completed system comprised 249 miles of sewers and cost £215,000. Initial attempts to connect water closets to the system failed because there was insufficient water available to flush the sewers properly (Liverpool had an intermittent water supply system until the mid-1860s).[38] Bristol, another unhealthy city, also installed an integrated sewerage system. By 1866, over 100 miles of main sewers had been constructed that emptied into the tidal Avon downriver from the city.[39] Bournemouth also took advantage of its coastal position to rid itself of its sewage. In 1885, *The Builder* reported the town had some 35 miles of sewers with three outlets into the sea.[40] For the size and complexity, no scheme could match the system of sewers designed for

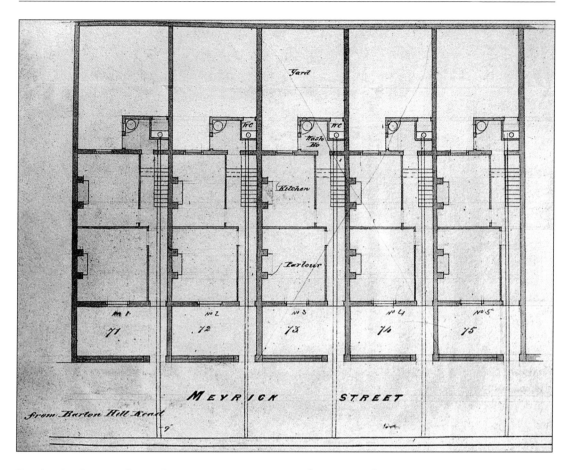

London by Sir Joseph Bazalgette (1819–91), the chief engineer of the Metropolitan Board of Works, established in 1856. Begun in 1859, this prodigious feat of civil engineering involved the laying of 1,300 miles of sewers and 82 miles of main intercepting sewers. These carried the sewage to great settlement tanks on the north bank of the Thames at Beckton and Crossness on the south bank from where it was pumped into the river just after high tide, ensuring that it did not flow back towards the city. The work continued until the 1870s, although the official opening by the Prince of Wales in April 1865 marked the official inauguration of the system.[41]

A plan of houses in Meyrick Street, Barton Hill, an industrial suburb of Bristol, 1875. The drawing shows the water closets in the backyards of these small terraced houses connected by a drain running under the house to the sewer in the street. (*Bristol Record Office*)

Where sewerage systems were installed connections from house drains to the sewers in the street were enforced by local boards of health. By 1859 in the two Clifton districts of Bristol, all but 844 of the 3,984 houses had been connected to the new sewer, while in the working-class district of Bedminster, 583 houses had been connected to the sewer completed in 1857.[42] At the same time, drain technology developed rapidly. The old cavernous drains made of porous brickwork, which often became blocked by accumulations of solid matter, were replaced by smaller more effective drains made of

Henry Doulton (1820–97)

H ENRY DOULTON was one of eight children born to John Doulton (1793–1873), who had joined a pottery in Vauxhall Walk, Lambeth in 1815. Henry joined his father's business in 1835, which was then trading as Doulton and Watts and located in Lambeth High Street. The company manufactured salt-glazed stoneware vessels, chiefly bottles for blacking, ink and beer. The younger Doulton rapidly acquired the skills of the potter and was soon playing a leading role in the running of the business. He introduced steam power for driving the throwing wheels, and by the late 1830s had begun manufacturing architectural terracotta and garden ornaments. To celebrate his coming of age, he produced a 300-gallon jar by hand, described as the largest stoneware vessel in the world.

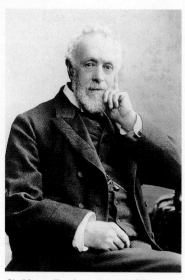

It was the opening of new works in Lambeth to manufacture salt-glazed stoneware sewer pipes in 1845 which was to transform the fortunes of the company and establish Henry Doulton's reputation. Edwin Chadwick, the leading sanitary reformer along with Doulton's friends, the engineering inspectors, Edward Cressy and Robert Rawlinson, convinced him that the stoneware pipe would form the basis of a sanitary revolution. The success of the new factory in Lambeth and the increasing demand for sanitary pipes led to the opening of additional factories at St Helen's in 1847 and Dudley in

Sir Henry Doulton. (*National Portrait Gallery*)

1848. By 1854, it was estimated that Doulton was responsible for a fifth of the sewer pipes produced in Great Britain. In 1854 John Watts retired and the company became known as Doulton and Co. Doulton manufactured his first ceramic sink in 1859, and by the 1860s was making stoneware closet pans. In 1877 Doulton entered a partnership with the old established firm of Pinder, Bourne and Co., at the Nile Street Pottery, Burslem, Stoke-on-Trent. They were important makers of tableware and earthenware sanitaryware. In 1882 Doulton gained complete control of the company and was able to consolidate his presence in the Potteries. In 1888 works were established in Paisley – primarily to manufacture cast-iron baths and cisterns – and production of fireclay goods at Dudley began in 1897.

By the 1890s Doulton and Co. were established as one of the leading sanitaryware manufacturers in Britain, but the company had, meanwhile, diversified into many other areas of ceramic manufacture, including art pottery and various types of tableware, including bone china. From the 1870s the company had been celebrated for its Lambeth 'faience', and in health exhibitions of the 1880s Doulton's stands often contained entire bathroom schemes featuring their own sanitary fittings and faience tilework. Doulton also staged impressive displays overseas, including the Philadelphia Centennial Exhibition of 1876 and the Chicago International Exhibition of 1893. Doulton was presented with the Albert Medal by the Royal Society of Arts in 1885 and knighted by Queen Victoria in 1887. The company continued to thrive after his death in 1897, and after a tortuous history of mergers in the twentieth century remains an important name in the field of bathroom ceramics.

impervious stoneware pipes. By concentrating the flow of water in a smooth circular channel its scouring power was increased. In the mid-1840s, Chadwick persuaded Henry Doulton (1820–1897), a Lambeth stoneware and terracotta manufacturer, to begin the manufacture of salt-glazed stoneware drainpipes. The venture was successful. It established Doulton's fortune and similar pipes were soon being made elsewhere. Gullies and traps of various kinds were also produced in stoneware while ventilators and covers for drains were made in cast-iron to make drains safer and more efficient.

The spread of water-carriage systems in towns encouraged the wider use of water closets. After several decades of limited use, the water closet was about to lose its exclusive middle-class image. In towns where integrated sewerage systems were installed, water closets became virtually a standard fitting in the typical working-class terraced house of between four and six rooms. In areas of back-to-back housing, they were sometimes contained in separate blocks built in the back lanes between rows of houses. In the case of through housing, where each dwelling had its own backyard, the closet was usually found in an outhouse reached from the yard. In working-class housing, therefore, the water closet was still separate from the main part of the house. Sophisticated valve and pan closets, however, were considered unsuitable for the poor as George Wilson, author of *Sanitary Hygiene*, observed in 1873: 'In the crowded districts of large towns, the ordinary form of wc has proved a failure partly on account of the complicated character of the contrivances for flushing but chiefly on account of the carelessness and filthy habits of the poorer classes.'[43] They were also too expensive. Some sort of simplified, cheap closet was required, therefore, for use by working-class families.

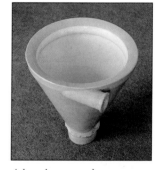

A long hopper and cottage pan – in cane and white ware. The pans were socketed on to a water-sealed trap, usually an S or shoot-down type. The long hopper (above) was originally installed in the outside facility of a villa residence built in Bristol in 1891 and the short hopper (below) comes from a house in Clevedon, north Somerset.

In 1845, the Revd Charles Girdlestone, rector of Alderley, Cheshire, and an active member of the Health of Towns Association, put forward his solution. He called it a 'soil-pan'. Nothing could be simpler. It consisted of a circular pan or basin attached to a water-sealed trap; there were no valves and no mechanics, therefore, to be abused by a careless user. Girdlestone illustrated one made of lead which had been in use for eighteen years – since about 1827 – although he had to admit that this was in the 'private' house of a gentleman.[44] The use of simple basins and traps appears to date from at least the start of the nineteenth century: a surviving Wedgwood pattern book of 1802, shows simple earthenware pans resembling deep funnels. J.C. Loudon illustrated something very similar in his *Cottage Farm and Villa Architecture* of 1833. This 'cheap basin and trap' was, he said, 'manufactured at the common tile potteries about London, and sold by retail at 2*s* 6*d*'.[45] Loudon's drawing suggests the bowl was made in one piece with the trap although they were usually in two parts.

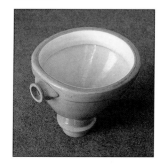

They were the first all-ceramic water closets, but were never exclusively a ceramic product. They were also made of cast iron, although as Girdlestone observed, this corroded over time, and then 'the filth is apt to adhere to it'.[46] By the 1850s iron founders had responded to this problem by lining the interiors of cast-iron basins with porcelain enamel.[47] Girdlestone illustrated another variant of the mid-1840s sold by Robert Wiss in Charing Cross, London, which consisted of a relatively shallow circular basin attached to a trap made of lead.[48] From the mid-nineteenth century fireclay came to be used for the manufacture of sanitaryware, and many basins and traps were made of a cheap fireclay known in the industry as cane and white ware: the exterior being the yellow-buff of the fireclay and the interior, a white ceramic glaze. There were also several variations according to the shape of the basin. The 'long hopper' was deep and straight-sided with a round rim, a shallower version was called the 'short hopper' and those with an oval and slightly rounded bowl were known as 'cottage' or 'servant's' closets. They were also named after the place where they were used: thus manufacturers made the 'Bristol Closet', the 'Liverpool Cottage Basin' and the 'Reading Pan' – but they were all very similar. Although Girdlestone and others could not have foreseen it, the all-ceramic pedestal closet – in other words, the modern 'toilet' – was ultimately developed out of this humble appliance.

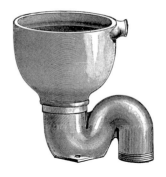

The 'Liverpool Cottage Basin' consisting of a round basin with a flushing rim set into an S trap. This one is from the 1895 catalogue of Sharpe Brothers and Co. The closet was available in cane and white ware and with an all-white basin which could be had with printed decoration. (*Sharpe Bros and Co. Ltd, Swadlincote*)

Robust and cheap, the simple basin and trap in its various guises – hopper and cottage pans – was seen by public-health reformers in the 1840s as the ideal water closet for use by the poor. In 1845 Girdlestone reported that in Huddersfield and other places – including Glasgow – soil pans had been introduced among the labouring classes. To support his argument, Girdlestone gave an instance of a house in Cross Street, Hatton Garden, London, which was let to six or seven working-class families. One pan had been fixed in the premises for the use of the house: he was informed it had answered 'most admirably'.[49] From the middle of the century, they were used extensively for working-class housing in towns which had invested in water-carriage systems. In larger houses, basin and trap closets were often provided for servant use. Distinctions of social class, therefore, were reinforced by the type of water closet used: expensive valve closets for the family and cheap basin and trap closets below stairs or behind the 'green baize door' of the service wing. The difference in price was marked. In 1884, the London sanitaryware manufacturers, Pontifex and Wood, advertised cottage pans and traps for as little as 3*s* 10*d*, while their cheapest Bramah valve closet cost £2 10*s*.[50]

Opinions as to the effectiveness of basin and trap water closets were mixed. 'In small dwellings with plenty of water, this closet answers its purpose admirably,' claimed J. Bailey Denton in 1876, but Walsh, in 1857, had not been so enthusiastic. He also emphasised the importance of a strong and plentiful flush of water, 'to carry the soil well out of the syphon bend', but added, 'in almost all cases where I have known it used there was an accumulation in the bend and some odour as a consequence of it'. Walsh, however, felt that the hopper –

'I have had one in use in my own house by my own family for the last fifteen years and it has served well.'
William Buchan on cottage closets, Glasgow, 1876.

or syphon closet as he called it – was 'sufficiently clean and wholesome' where it opened to external air, but too smelly to be used indoors.[51] The problem was that hopper and cottage closets were usually denied the quantity of flush water they required to clear the waste. Sometimes they were denied it altogether. They were frequently installed in poorer housing without a connection to a cistern: the only way the closet could be flushed was by throwing a bucket of water into the pan, but this could also result in the trap losing its water through syphonic action. But where the vessel was connected to a cistern, the flush water was rarely strong enough to clean it. Long hopper pans with their deep sides were the worst, and writing of them in 1891, Hellyer pointed out how the long, tapering sides of the interior provided a large surface area on which excrement would stick: it was difficult for this to be removed by such a weak flushing action. 'The water enters the closet,' he explained, 'with such a twirling motion that by the time it has twirled itself down to the trap, it has no energy left to carry anything with it; and so it just gravitates through the drain to the sewer, leaving matters in the closet pretty much as it had found them.'[52] Hellyer's verdict was that as water closets, hoppers were useless. But he did suggest another use to which they could be put: 'Instead of destroying the thousands already made, they might be used by market gardeners for protecting certain things from frost, as rhubarb.' Nevertheless, hopper and cottage closets were still on sale twenty years later.[53]

So hopper and cottage basins were often found in a filthy state. While the inadequacies of the design and the installation may have been the root cause, some reformers were inclined to blame the occupants. Poor people with dirty habits, as Wilson and others pointed out, could not be relied upon to use an appliance properly – least of all flush it after use. The responsibility, therefore, had to be taken out of their hands, the flushing arranged by an automatic contrivance or by an operative – a scavenger or caretaker. One solution was the trough closet. This device was shown in J.C. Morton's *Cyclopaedia of Agriculture*, published in 1855. It consisted of a series of closets placed over a trough or tank kept half full with water which sloped to one side where a large plug enabled it to be periodically emptied into a cesspit. It was recommended for the cottages of agricultural labourers where it was located in an outhouse in the yard.[54] The following year a similar arrangement featured in the catalogue

'The rich have no easy task to keep their water closets in order – so how would the ignorant, the poor and the careless who form the vast majority of town populations cope?'
James Hole, 1866.

A trough closet, by John Warner and Sons, Cripplegate, London, 1856. The underground tank was supplied with water from the supply on the left and flushed once or twice a day by pulling the plug that is just visible in the murk on the right.

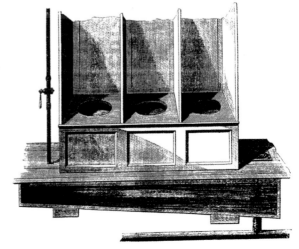

of the London brass founders, John Warner and Sons.[55] They showed a three-seat version divided by vertical partitions, 'recommended for the use of schools, unions [workhouses], asylums and other public establishments where no care is required to ensure their efficiency'. The closet was designed to be flushed just once or twice a day by pulling up a handle sunk in the floor using a rod or chain. This handle was connected to the plug in the bottom of the tank by a vertical rod and once emptied, clean water could be swilled through from a tap at the side and the tank refilled. As the closet was used through the day, the water in the tank, visible through the seat hole, turned to raw, liquid sewage: in warm weather the stench must have been unbearable.

Trough closets were adopted for use in the crowded courts of Liverpool where, in the 1870s, they were regarded as superior to 'what are called water closets in the poor neighbourhoods of London and other large towns'.[56] Across the Mersey in Birkenhead, the tumbler closet was preferred. These were similar to trough closets in consisting of a series of closets, but were flushed by a swinging tank gradually filled by a constant trickle of water. When the tank was almost full it capsized and the contents of the trough flushed into the drain. They were also used in Leeds, and from 1887, James Duckett of Burnley, Lancashire, combined tipping tanks with individual closets, known as 'tipper closets'.* Trough and tumbler closets were favoured for removing the responsibility of flushing from the user, but as the flow of water was also strictly controlled, they also probably won the approval of water companies concerned with excessive consumption of water in closets.

Eventually, trough closets were condemned as insanitary – along with pan closets and hopper pans. In Liverpool, trough closets were gradually phased out – there were only 1,459 left by 1905. But at least the problem of where the waste went beyond the pan had been resolved. In 1873, Wilson said that removal by water was the only system suited for large towns.[57] By the mid-1870s, Leicester had joined the list of towns on the water-carriage system along with Croydon, Bedford and Leamington Spa.[58] By 1878 Robert Rawlinson in his book *Sanitary Science* reckoned that in London there were about 700,000 water closets in use: that was about one closet to one in five people.[59] But not everyone was convinced that discharging sewage in the crude state into the Thames estuary, the Mersey and close to beaches at Bournemouth – and elsewhere – was desirable. The debate raged for several decades and was to have a major bearing on the development of sanitary fittings.

'In the north of England, this kind of closet is much used and is reported to be well adapted for poor neighbourhoods.'
William Eassie on trough closets, 1872.

---

* See chapter eight.

CHAPTER THREE

Perfectly Sweet and Wholesome
dry privies and earth closets

The construction of new sewerage systems in London and other towns and cities that adopted the water-carriage system represented a massive feat of Victorian civil engineering. Reporting on sanitary improvements at the International Exhibition held in London in 1862, Dr Angus Smith claimed, 'we may consider it certain that no plan will ever be devised for removing refuse from our houses equal to an underground flow, self-acting and out of sight'.[1] But not everyone was so sure. In 1863, the trade journal *The Ironmonger* replied, 'there is something radically wrong in the plan which Dr Angus Smith extols for it leads to the pollution of our rivers with matter which might be used to fertilise our lands'.[2]

The fertilising value of human waste had long been recognised. Every year large quantities of nightsoil were shipped by barge from London for use on the land. But the arrival of the water-carriage system after 1850 concentrated people's minds anew on the subject, and in the 1850s and 1860s, the idea that town sewage could be utilised as manure attracted widespread support. In 1851, by which time the idea of intercepting sewers for London had been aired, Henry Mayhew wrote of 'the folly, not to say wickedness' of discharging liquid sewage into the River Thames. A large proportion of the capital's drinking water at the time came from the Thames, prompting Mayhew to further reflect, 'we import guano and drink a solution of our own faeces'.[3] Mayhew was not alone. In 1853, John Joseph Mechi (1801–80), who promoted progressive agricultural methods on his farm at Tiptree, Essex, likened sewage running to waste as a 'stream of liquid guano'.[4] Mechi, a successful London businessman, who had turned to farming in 1841, was influenced by the theories of Justus von Liebig (1803–73), professor of chemistry at Giessen University. In his book *Agricultural Chemistry*, published in 1861, Liebig wrote, 'the introduction of water closets into most parts of England results in the loss annually

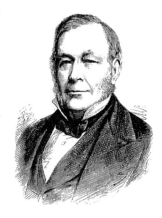

John Joseph Mechi (1801–80) had amassed a fortune as a cutler in Leadenhall Street, London, selling his patent razor strops. He turned to farming and became an active supporter of the utilisation of sewage on the land.

of the materials capable of producing food for three and a half million people'.[5]

Advances in agricultural science from the 1830s and 1840s had stimulated the demand for imported fertilisers such as Peruvian guano, first imported in about 1847, and animal bone, while the manufacture of superphosphates – the first artificial fertiliser – commenced in 1842. 'Men of middle age,' wrote P.H. Frere in 1863, 'who have watched the rise and progress of the entire market for artificial manures will recollect that, when guano first appeared, bones and soot were almost the only auxiliaries of farmyard manure in common use.'[6] While farmers were spending more on these new fertilisers, municipal authorities were grappling with the problem of disposing of huge quantities of human excrement from their rapidly expanding populations. Could the two issues be linked? There were many who believed they were, and for several decades, agricultural and sanitary science found a common cause which was to take the development of the closet in a new direction.

A common cause, however, could only be established if the value of town sewage as a farm manure was confirmed scientifically. John Bennet Lawes (1814–1900), who had established an experimental farm at Rothampstead, Hertfordshire in the 1830s, was convinced that the agricultural value of human sewage could offset the value of its disposal. Aided by his scientific assistant, Henry Gilbert (1817–1901), Lawes studied samples of sewage collected in Rugby between 1861 and 1863 for the Royal Commission on the Sewage of Towns established in 1857. They concluded that of the 60 or so tons of dilute sewage generated per inhabitant per year, 12½ lb consisted of ammonia which was equivalent in manurial terms to about 74 lb of guano. With imported guano priced at £12 a ton in the early 1860s, this established the value of the annual sewage of one person at about 8*s*.[7] A slightly higher figure for London sewage was provided by Professor Way to a Parliamentary Select Committee set up in 1864 to 'Enquire into any plans for Dealing with the Sewage of the Metropolis and other Large Towns, with a View to its Utilisation for Agricultural Purposes'. Professor Way reckoned that the annual value of the sewage in the capital was equivalent to 10*s* 6*d* per person.[8] In the light of such calculations, extravagant claims were made of the savings which could be made by using town sewage on the land. One estimate even reckoned that the annual value of the waste of the entire population would halve the interest on the national debt.[9]

Nevertheless, the general conclusion of the Royal Commission was that sewage disposal on farmland was unlikely to generate any significant income for towns, but could be of social benefit.

'The insanitary evils which have occurred to the health of the population by the introduction of underground or subterranean drains are incalculable. . . .'
Dr Chesshire to the Royal Society of Arts, 1878.

Notwithstanding this cautious verdict, the last quarter of the nineteenth century saw upwards of 100 large towns and cities launch schemes for the distribution of their sewage as farm manure. As early as 1853 Mechi had envisaged a system where liquid sewage would be conducted to farms through pipes and then hosed on to individual fields. In 1864 the Metropolitan Board of Works approved a scheme devised by William Hope and William Napier to convey the sewage from the north bank of the Thames by a 44-mile culvert to reclaim land on the Maplin Sands in Essex. Hope had estimated the scheme would yield a profit before interest of £365,000.[10] After considerable initial optimism, the project faltered through lack of capital and was never finished, but elsewhere schemes to irrigate farms with town sewage were carried through to completion. In 1871 the corporation of Leamington Spa inaugurated a system which pumped liquid sewage to Heathcote Farm, owned by the Earl of Warwick, about 2 miles from the town centre. In Reading, the corporation established two municipally run farms supplied with sewage from about 30,000 of the town's inhabitants. A handsome pumping station was built at Blake's Lock on the River Kennet to pipe sewage to the farms.[11]

These municipally sponsored sewage farms only confirmed the findings of the Royal Commission – that there was little money to be made out of muck – at least in the liquid state. The problem, quite simply, was that the modest income it yielded as farm manure did not cover the substantial capital investment involved in laying the sewers and constructing the means of distribution to individual farms. The manurial content of the sewage was also diluted by the huge quantities of nutritionless water carried with it. Moreover, water-carriage systems were not only expensive but could also be troublesome. Writing in 1863, the Revd Henry Moule (1801–80), vicar of Fordington, Dorset, cited the case of Birmingham, where, he said, 'the great outlay and the perplexities which have arisen from partial and unsuccessful attempts to carry out the water closet system . . . has involved the town in endless troubles and litigations'. The alternative solution promoted by Moule and many others was to keep the excrement dry. The same year, John Lawes was quoted in *The Ironmonger* as conceding that the productiveness of agricultural land, 'devoted to the growth of human food' might be increased if a system was devised which would, 'preserve the excrements of the population free from admixture with water'.[12] These were the measured words of a farmer steeped in agricultural science – for the evangelical Moule, who saw most things in life in black and white, sewage was a 'great national evil', an evil that had to be eradicated.[13]

The Revd Henry Moule (1801–1880)

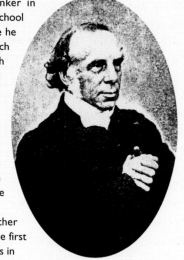

The Revd Henry Moule.

HENRY MOULE was the sixth son of a solicitor and banker in Melksham, Wiltshire. He attended Marlborough Grammar School and graduated from Cambridge in 1821. While at Cambridge he came under the influence of the Evangelical movement, which became one of the most important influences on Victorian life. Although deeply conservative and puritanical, Evangelists were also concerned with social reform. Moule entered the Church and in 1829 became Rector of Fordington, near Dorchester in Dorset, where he found immense physical, moral and social problems, with many villagers living in wretched accommodation in appalling sanitary conditions. Moule's puritanical views initially made him very unpopular, but this changed following his selfless devotion to the villagers during two outbreaks of cholera in 1849 and 1854, and from the 1860s there was a religious revival in the parish. Moule was determined that something radical must be done to improve conditions, especially the supply of water and sanitary arrangements.

In 1859 he took out his first patent for evaporating sewage and other waters, and patented his earth closet in 1860. Although Moule was not the first to patent a dry closet his device enjoyed considerable success, and this was in no small part due to his energy and business acumen. He believed firmly in the value of his earth-closet manure at a time when the dry system of sewage disposal attracted influential support. He also took out patents for heating hothouses by passing steam into a chamber below the beds and for fuelling locomotives with a mixture of powdered coal, oil and limestone. He also devised an apparatus for heating churches and schoolrooms and developed a phospho-silicon manure in collaboration with a neighbour, William Allardyce. Moule, who was a friend of the novelist, Thomas Hardy, and a distant relative of the diarist, the Revd Francis Kilvert, had eight children by his wife, Mary. One died in infancy, but several went on to lead distinguished lives. He was also a friend of the Dorset dialect poet, William Barnes, and with him and another founded the Dorset Museum in 1845.

Moule had the answer. For him it was a matter of earth versus water and in 1860 he obtained patent protection for a dry closet which used dry and sifted earth to absorb what he called the 'excrementitious and other offensive matter' to make manure. Moule had started by experimenting with his own household at the vicarage in Fordington. He blocked up the existing cesspool and replaced it with buckets which were emptied from 'time to time' and mixed with garden soil. 'The removal and mixing,' he explained, 'only occupied a boy's time for a quarter of an hour and after all was completed, within ten minutes, neither eye nor nose could perceive anything offensive.'[14] He then discovered that if the soil was stored under cover it could be re-used up to five times before it lost its absorbent powers. The disintegration of the faeces was caused by bacteria naturally occurring in the soil. About 1½lb of soil, it was found, was required to deodorise one stool. The type of soil was also important: rich garden soil was best, then peaty soils; sandy loams and sand were the least effective.[15] Moule's closet was not suitable for disposing of urine and household slops. These had to be removed either by pouring them into drains or a pit in the garden.

Moule's earth closet was adapted according to the means of the householder. For a cottager, he recommended that the vault or pit in the cottage garden was filled in and replaced with a square enclosure of brick or stone under the seat. The base was to be watertight and placed just a few inches below the floor of the privy. An opening at the back of the enclosure enabled the earth to be removed when necessary. Round the back of the privy he recommended that a 'rough shed' was built to store a cartload of earth. The shed would have two compartments either side of the entrance, each being used alternately as the wet and dry store. Used this way, Moule estimated that one load of earth would be enough for two or three people for between six and twelve months.[16]

For 'better homes and larger establishments' Moule designed several self-contained mechanical earth closets, three versions of which were described in his patent. One design was to be made with a movable base that tipped when the closet handle was pulled. In theory, the excrement and powdered earth would slide off the base into a cavity below. When the base swung back to the horizontal with the aid of a spring or counterbalance, a simple mechanism caused a rotary feeder behind the seat to make a quarter turn, tipping fresh earth on to the base in readiness for the next use. Another arrangement illustrated in the patent consisted of a trough under the seat which contained a rotating axle, turned through bevel gearing from a crank handle beside the seat, which was designed to thoroughly mix the excrement and earth. A third version was

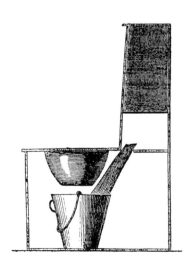
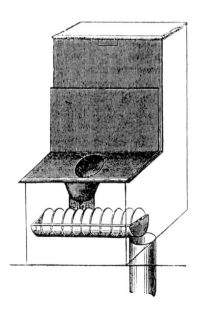

Two of Moule's earth closets manufactured by James White and Co., Dorchester in 1863. Both had fixed pans below the seat. The pan of the closet on the left had a movable base which rotated upwards against the sides so that the waste was scraped into the bucket or void below. With a conventional lifting handle, this closet cost £2 7s 6d. The version on the right was fitted with a screw rotating in a trough to mix the various constituents of the waste; it was almost twice as expensive.

supplied with a container with a rounded bottom which swung upwards when the closet handle was pulled: the bottom edge of the side casing acting as a scraper.

Moule soon arranged for James White and Co. of 45 High East Street in Dorchester to manufacture his earth closets. By 1863, they were producing two versions similar to two of the designs featured in the patent, although the type with the trough was fitted with a revolving screw in place of separate blades which, Moule explained, ensured that paper was torn to pieces and a 'thorough mixture effected'.[17] They were soon being made by other makers including the Bristol brass founders, Llewellins and James[18] and John Parker in Woodstock, Oxfordshire, who, advertising his earth closets in 1873 claimed that 'they keep the place perfectly sweet and wholesome'.[19] By the mid-1860s, the closets were also being made by Moule's Earth Closet Co., Covent Garden, London, with J.W. Girdlestone as its engineer. In 1873 Moule and Girdlestone patented an improved closet which had a hopper at the back connected to the closet handle by a lever: when the handle was pulled the hopper was drawn forward releasing a quantity of earth into a conventional iron bucket under the seat.[20]

Moule's earth closet was a success and widely adopted from the 1860s. By 1863, the system was being used at the workhouse school in Bradford on Avon, Wiltshire, where there were fifty-five children. The vice chairmen of the Board of Guardians found that after five months, the whole compost did not exceed a cartload and a half and that there was nothing offensive, unlike the previous arrangements, where 'all had been noxious pungency'.[21] They were introduced in other workhouses and in some prisons. In 1866, Captain Armytage, the governor of Wakefield prison, West Yorkshire, introduced the system, and by 1872 there were 776 in use within the prison.[22] They

Left: Moule's 'pull-up' earth closet, patented in 1873. Largely unaltered, this closet was still on sale in the 1930s. *Right:* Improved self-acting earth closet sold by the Reading Iron Co., *c.* 1905. When the closet was used the seat was depressed forcing down the vertical rods connected to a toothed lever. The teeth of the lever engaged with those of a similar lever connected to a sliding shovel at the base of the storage box containing the dry earth. When the seat was depressed the shovel was forced up and backwards under the earth and when the seat was relieved, it was quickly pulled forward spreading earth over the excreta in the bucket. The storage box held sufficient earth for fifty uses of the closet.

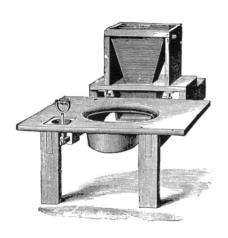
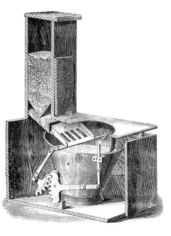

were a success. The prison was rid of overpowering smells and each year some 50 to 60 tons of earth manure was obtained and used in the prison grounds with 'remarkable success' in the growing of onions and other vegetables. If the distribution and collection of the earth was labour-intensive, this was hardly a problem: prisoners were used. Warders were permitted to take up to five inmates to the earth shed for exchanging the pans. Earth closets were also adopted by large agricultural landlords on their estates. Lord Wantage, for example, who rebuilt the two villages of Ardington and East Lockinge on his Berkshire estate from the 1860s, built new cottages for the estate workers which were equipped with sheds at the back containing earth closets.[23]

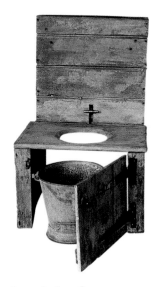

An earth closet from a cottage at Coalpit Heath, South Gloucestershire, which was used until the late 1950s. Pulling the brass handle behind the seat released the earth which fell into the special galvanised iron bucket under the seat.

A detailed description of the operation of earth closets on a large country estate survives in a report drawn up by Sir Anthony de Rothschild's land agent at Halton, Buckinghamshire.[24] The agent made a personal inspection of the scheme in the mid-1870s, by which time about 170 to 180 earth closets supplied by Moule's Earth Closet Co. were installed in the farmhouses and cottages on the estate. The system required about 200 tons of earth annually which was dug and sifted in dry weather. It was stored in a large open shed and dried over a giant 'hot plate' – a thick iron sheet, 9 ft square – heated by a fire and flues running underneath. One man – a 'scavenger'– was employed to maintain the closets. Two or three times a week he took a cartload of dried earth around the estate, filling the hoppers and, if necessary, levelling the soil in the vaults under the seat. These were then emptied at intervals ranging from six weeks to three months depending on the use of the closet. After the first use, the soil was taken to the shed and heated and dried and then redistributed to the closets. After the second use it was collected and stored and eventually used as agricultural manure. 'The closets,' reported Rothschild's agent, 'are not expensively built, but they are well attended to. They are patterns of decency and cleanliness. Not the least smell of any kind was perceptible except where the vaults are not water tight, and they, of course, approximate very nearly to the condition of the common privy.'

Moule was keen to see other rural landlords introduce the earth system on their estates believing it would lead to the greater 'comfort, contentment and prosperity of the working classes'.[25] He wrote extensively of its benefits – that it was healthier and more economical than the water-closet system – being cheaper to install and producing a valuable end product in the form of manure. Moule had witnessed the effects of cholera in his parish, and although various theories as to its causes were still current, he was clearly aware of the fatal connection between dirt and disease. 'The health of towns,' he declared in 1863, 'may be promoted by the entire removal of the sewage nuisance.'[26] Moule was also aware of the value of the earth closet in rural areas that often had a higher rate of mortality than London and other 'first rate towns', which, by the 1860s were becoming healthier places to live. Moule was extremely critical of the expense of the water-carriage system. He gave examples of the savings that could be made in schools and prisons if his earth closets replaced the use of water closets. 'The truth is,' he wrote in 1863, 'that the machinery is more simple, much less expensive and far less liable to injury than that of the water closet.' He claimed that the expense of installing an earth closet was about a quarter that of a water closet. And then there was the case of Birmingham where Moule condemned the expense – some £26,000 – incurred in buying land and constructing two high-level sewers and tanks to form part of a water-carriage system. Here Moule was not alone, and as late as 1878 others in Birmingham remained deeply critical of the adoption of water closets in the city. Like the proponents of sewage irrigation, Moule also calculated the powers of the used soil as manure. He cited cases where better vegetables and crops were cultivated as a result of applying the earth to cottage gardens and fields. He described the success with which a cottager in Blandford, Dorset adopted the system in his large garden in the spring of 1862. The cottager applied the manure to patches of mangold and swedes and the land steward who had initially persuaded him to try the system told the vicar 'he never saw such fine roots as were grown'.[27] Convinced by this and other examples, Moule claimed the used earth was as effective as superphosphates in promoting the growth of turnips, and with an eye to its monetary value reckoned a ton of used earth could be valued at £3 10*s* if it was recycled seven times.[28]

Moule's energy, conviction and business acumen clearly contributed to the success of his earth closet after 1860, but he was not the first to patent a dry closet. Three years earlier, in June 1857, a medical doctor from Llangefui in Anglesey, John Lloyd, invented a dry disposal system, similar in many respects to Moule's but with one fundamental difference: Lloyd's deodorising material was not earth but the ordinary refuse of fireplaces: cinders and ash. The faeces were acted upon by the addition of 'fresh ashes' – that is, perfectly dry ash – which, he said, 'rapidly solidifies and even fossilises the faeces and converts them to dry masses or cakes, without any smells which can be compressed, pounded or packed, as may be desired'. The ashes could, if necessary, be supplemented by quicklime. Lloyd's closet was supplied with a portable, square metal container under the seat to collect the waste. It was divided by a curved partition which separated the faeces from the urine as they fell – 'a circumstance', the

doctor explained, 'depending entirely upon anatomical consider-
ations, and which acts in the case of women as well as men'.[29]

Lloyd's simplest arrangement involved the use of a ladle to apply
the ash, but his patent also specified a wooden closet, like a
commode, made with a storage box or feeder above and behind the
seat. A grating was placed over the urine compartment at the front of
the container to prevent paper falling in, while a 'valve' covered the
rear half to prevent liquids from entering and 'noxious smells from
rising'. The valve, consisting of a large board or sheet, was operated
by a conventional closet handle or a self-acting mechanism activated
by rising from the seat. Two cog wheels connected the valve to a
revolving cylinder at the base of the hopper. This was made with
projections forming individual pockets which fed some of the ash
into the rear half of the container. The urine compartment was
prepared in advance with layers of lime and ash. Moule's mechanical
earth closet, patented three years later was very similar. Lloyd also
anticipated Moule in believing that his system could be organised for
entire communities with dry ash stored in depots and like Moule was
certain the dry sewage constituted a saleable commodity.

Following Lloyds's patent and before Moule was granted his in
1860, several patents for dry closets were granted. The success of
Moule's earth closet has eclipsed these earlier initiatives but it is
possible that Moule drew on the information contained in these
existing patents to create his own system. Alternatively, the
Fordington vicar may have found his inspiration in the Old
Testament, where, in Deuteronomy, Moses laid down that human
waste should be buried in earth. Whatever the source of the idea,
Moule's success lay in his ability to turn it into a commercial success.
There is no evidence that Lloyd ever put his device into practice,
although his patent established several features that were to become
basic to many dry closets. His patent created the commode-like
appearance of free-standing dry closets with earth supplied from a
hopper at the back with the aid of a simple mechanism. Lloyd also
understood the importance of keeping the waste dry, and many
patents were taken out over the following decades for dry closets
which separated the urine from the faeces. This became known as the
dry or conservancy system – the drainage being restricted to waste
water. The other important feature was the use of ash as the
deodorising material.

Many ingenious – but not always practical – suggestions for
alternative deodorising substances were made. One was charcoal
which was used in dry closets in Leeds and elsewhere, but proved too
expensive to be used on a large scale.[30] Other materials which appear

'And thou shalt have a paddle upon thy weapon; and it shall be, when thou wilt ease thyself abroad, thou shalt dig therewith, and shalt turn back and cover that which cometh from thee.'
Deuteronomy 23: 13.

in patents include wood shavings and horn clippings, but they would have had little absorbent or deodorising power. The recommended use of waste industrial products such as coal tar, soap boilers' waste and used bark from tanneries can only have represented an attempt to replace one evil smell with another. Several patents suggested the use of road sweepings including horse droppings: this plentiful material was used to make bricks and added by builders to plaster, but it was a curious notion that animal dung could be used to neutralise the human variety. But the one waste material that every Victorian town had in abundance was cinders and ash from domestic fires. It was generated in large quantities by virtually every urban household. Writing in 1851, Mayhew reckoned some 3,500,000 tons of coal was burned per annum in London producing a vast amount of ash and cinders which had to be removed by dust contractors. This was one deodorising agent, therefore, that did not require delivering: it was already on site; moreover, it cost nothing and at its source – the hearth or ash pit – was dry and perfectly odourless. John Conyers Morrell, from Leyland, Lancashire, an inventor and manufacturer of ash closets, went further and argued that ash was the equal of dried earth as a deodorant and superior as an absorbent.[31]

The combination of ash pits – where household cinders and ash were dumped – and the privy-midden was an established feature of many northern towns in the nineteenth century. The ash was thrown into an enclosed space below and behind the privy seat where it soaked up the liquid in the waste. This was the dry privy – the 'netty' to the Newcastle Geordie – and was adopted with detail differences by many local authorities as a cheap alternative to the

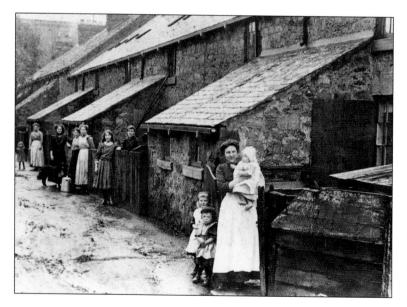

The front row of back-to-back colliery houses at Twizell, near Morpeth, Northumberland, *c*. 1900. The 'netties' or privies were contained in the lean-to structures at the front. (*Beamish, The North of England Open Air Museum*)

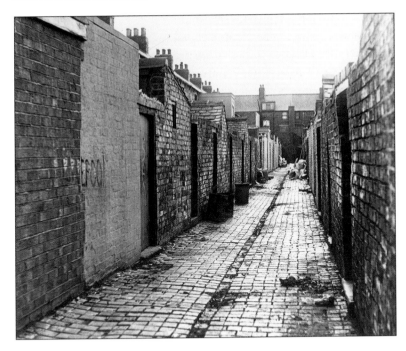

Former dry privies in the back lane between rows of terraced houses in Middlesbrough, photographed in 1979. The back alleys provided access for the municipal dustmen to remove the waste. (*Beamish, The North of England Open Air Museum*)

water-carriage system. It was essential the ash was kept dry or the arrangement was no better than the old 'wet' privy with its cesspool. So the ash pit was enclosed or covered over in some way and made reasonably watertight. In Preston, Leeds and Birmingham, according to George Wilson in 1873, the pits were large – with correspondingly large accumulations of waste – but they were compulsorily covered over. In Manchester, the pits were lined with Rochdale flags set in mortar and had a bottom sloping to an outlet opening into a drain. The ashes and other house refuse were added through an opening in the front of the privy seat or by lifting the seat where it was hinged. The arrangement was similar in Hull, except the midden was reduced to the space under the seat. In Hull, the ashes were thrown through a hole in the seat and the front board was removable so the scavenger could take away the contents.[32] Sanitarians such as Wilson considered the smaller pits were preferable as they had to be emptied more frequently. Nevertheless, Wilson added, 'even when it is carried out with every regard to structural detail and management, the midden system will always be objectionable, not only on account of the great expense of scavenging, but also because of the annoyance and discomfort necessarily arising from the frequent visitations of the soil cart'.[33]

In some of the dry privies in Manchester, according to Wilson, the ash was thrown into a chute provided with an iron grid which sifted the cinders from the ashes so they could be used again. Some of the grids were made to shake the ash with the aid of a simple mechanical

'I believe that no known or projected system yet has been found to answer the requirements of a large or small town equal to the Lancashire ash pit.' Mr Wallworth, Manchester Scavengers' Department, 1864.

device. The first patent for a mechanical cinder sifter was taken out by J.S. Dawes in 1859.[34] Then in 1866, John Conyers Morrell took out the first of eight patents for dry closets. They were made by Morrell's own Sanitary Appliance Co. in Manchester and most contained a self-acting mechanical cinder sifter. The system required no extra effort on the part of the householder: the house ashes were simply thrown through a hole in the side of the closet if it was a self-contained unit or through a hole in the wall if fitted into the privy structure. The cinders and ash landed on a riddle or sieve placed at an angle about 4 ft above the ground at the back of the closet. The riddle was agitated by a self-acting device triggered by rising from the seat or closing the privy door. The fine ash passed through the wire mesh to a chute and then into the 'manure receptacle' while the cinders rolled off the top of the sieve to a store at the back of the closet. They could then be re-used as fuel or used to filter household slops and urine before these liquids were let into the drains.

The fine ash, meanwhile, thoroughly deodorised the excrement which then formed a valuable farm or garden manure. Like other exponents of the dry system, Morrell was keen to emphasise the economy of his system. He claimed the cost of application was not

'Your Morrell's patent cinder sifting ash closet which was placed in my backyard about twelve months ago has given me great satisfaction.'
Dr Eyton Jones,
Wrexham, 1901.

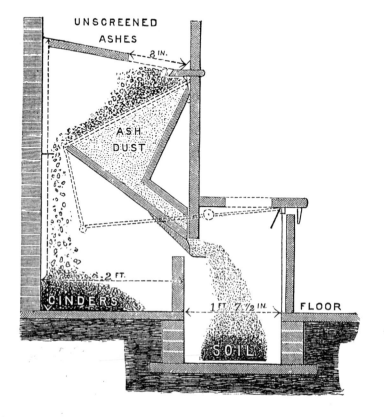

UNSCREENED
ASHES

2 IN.

ASH
DUST

2 FT.

CINDERS

1 FT. 7 1/2 IN.   FLOOR

SOIL

From 1867, J. Conyers Morrell introduced several types of cinder-sifting dry privy which were made in Manchester by his Sanitary Appliance Co. A simple mechanical device usually operated by depressing the seat shook a wire mesh riddle that sifted the fine ash from the household cinders. The ash then dropped by a chute into the receptacle containing the waste. Morrell patented this particular closet in 1884.

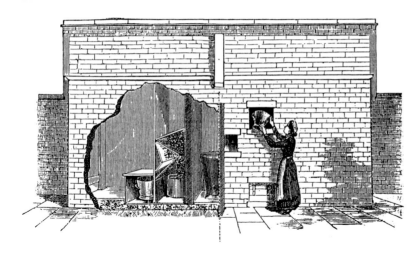

The Manchester pail system, 1883. This double privy is seen from the house; the doors are at each side. Ashes are thrown through a hatch onto a riddle where the fine dust falls into the pail under the seat while the cinders fall into another pail to be re-used as fuel. Dustmen removed the filled buckets through hatches on the other side.

greater than the old midden system and much less than that of the water closet.[35] His first patent of 1866 described how the deodorised human excrement could be carried in 'suitable closed carts' to a building containing several drying floors, heated by steam or hot-water pipes for further drying and preparing the waste as manure.[36] Morrell's closets attracted considerable interest at sanitary exhibitions from the 1870s; a half-sized working model of one was displayed at the International Health Exhibition in 1884, and the following year one was awarded a prize at the Sanitary Institute's eighth congress at Leicester.[37] Cinder sifting ash closets were adopted on a large scale in the Pendleton area of Salford. By the mid-1870s more than 1,000 closets were in use in the district producing 3,900 tons of crude manure per annum. The waste was collected in pails containing 1½ cwt and conveyed in covered vans to manure works constructed by the corporation at Windsor Bridge and alongside the canal. Using steam-powered mills, the 'excrementitious' matter was mixed with sulphate of lime, producing a 'consolidated manure of uniform consistency'. This was then sold at 12*s* 6*d* per ton. Hard material such as cinders was ground in a second mill and sold for use in mortar. The annual profit to the corporation was £1,475 3*s*.[38] So providing it was kept dry, perhaps there was money – or 'brass' – to be made out of muck?

The simplest dry disposal system consisted of nothing more than a bucket: to the Victorian sanitarian this was the 'pail system'. In 1876 J. Bailey Denton stated, 'middens with removable receptacles such as are now coming into use in Manchester and other northern towns form an improvement on the old privy or midden system. They allow of the ready removal of the excreta, and as the receptacles are of a comparatively small size, they luckily necessitate frequent

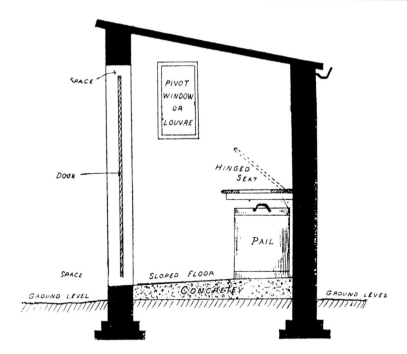

A pail closet of 1892. The pail is covered by a hinged seat with a hole resting on two side brackets. There is no front panel, although many were made with an enclosed seat.

emptying.'[39] By the mid-1870s, the pail system was in operation in many Midland and northern towns including Birmingham, Nottingham, Rochdale, Blackburn, and Warrington. The container was usually nothing more than a disused cask, sawn in half or a galvanised iron bucket. A sprinkling of ash or some other material was sometimes added to the container to absorb the liquid and deodorise the solid contents, although in Leeds, according to George Wilson in 1873, the boxes used were given no preparation.[40] The other important practical requirement was regular emptying. As Denton emphasised in 1876, 'in all towns and villages, where a dry system of excrement removal is adopted, it is essentially necessary that this duty should be performed by one man under the orders of the sanitary authority, and not left to individual performance'.[41] Individual performance, in fact, was not to be trusted. In 1878 at the third annual conference on the Health and Sewage of Towns organised by the Royal Society of Arts, J.M. Fox, the medical officer of health for mid-Cheshire said, 'dirty and inconsiderate people will foul and spoil the best arrangements. Such persons', he continued, 'must undergo a course of correction and education.'[42]

Rochdale provided a model of how the pail system could be operated to ensure that the vessels were routinely emptied and replaced and how the waste could be recycled. In this Lancashire mill town with a population in the 1870s of about 71,000, the collection of excreta pails and ash tubs was organised by dividing the town into

'. . . dirty and inconsiderate people will foul the best arrangements. Such persons must undergo a course of correction and education.'

J.M. Fox, Medical Officer of Health for Mid-Cheshire, 1878.

six districts so that the weekly collection of every individual pail or tub could be monitored. In 1876, Denton described how the system worked.

> Vans and ash-carts are appropriated for the collection, and the guard is furnished every morning with the names of the streets and number of closets in that street, written on a ruled blank list, which he has to collect. When the van or cart returns it is weighed, and the list given to the weigh clerk, in the ruled squares of which the guard has entered the pail or ash tub number . . . an inspector daily enters from these lists into the division book the numbers of pails brought in, and is thus able to say at the close of the week if every closet has been attended to.

The ash carts tipped their contents into a sifting machine which separated the fine ash from cinders, rags, vegetables and other hard waste. The cinders were recovered and used for the steam boilers at the works, the clinker and pots ground up for mortar and cement while the rags, glasses and iron were sold. The excrement and urine from the pails was emptied into a trench filled with fine ash obtained from the sifted cinders. Sulphuric acid was poured into the trench and the whole mixed. After being left for three weeks, dug over and screened the waste was sold as manure. The pails, meanwhile, were then thoroughly washed and a quantity of aluminium chloride and calcium sulphate added to desiccate the waste when the pails were next used.[43] The town adopted the system in about 1868, and in 1870 there were 527 pails in use: by 1878, the figure had risen to 7,504 with 1,200 old privies and middens remaining. The result was that Rochdale became a healthier place to live in: according to a local doctor the death rate of the town dropped from 27 to 21 per 1,000 between 1870 and 1878.[44]

The pail system worked best – or was least offensive – when some sort of dry deodorising material or absorbent was placed in the bucket. The Goux Absorbent Pail System, patented by a Frenchman, Pierre Goux, in 1868,[45] involved lining the interior of the tubs variously with chaff, straw or stable litter, loft sweepings, spent tan or hops or even dry ferns, in other words, with virtually any dry waste readily to hand. To this a little soot, charcoal, gypsum (calcium sulphate) or other deodoriser was added.[46] The mixture was packed firmly in the pails using a mould – apparently one boy

'I would at once give it as my opinion that the absorbent packing of the Goux system answers the great end of arresting decomposition'. Dr Goldie, Medical Officer of Health for Leeds, *c.* 1883.

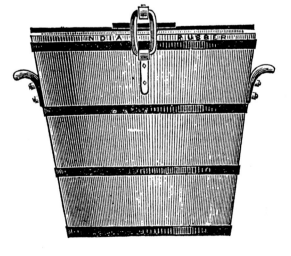

A Rochdale pail fitted with Haresceugh's sprung lid, patented in 1876, which was provided with an india-rubber cushion so the pail was hermetically sealed when collected. In the early 1880s Rochdale replaced iron with wooden pails as they were cheaper, lasted longer and could be more easily repaired.

could pack eighty an hour – and was supposed to be sufficiently absorbent for urine to be emptied into the tub. By the mid-1870s, over 3,000 of Goux's closets were in use in Halifax, reducing the quantity of raw liquid sewage which drained into the River Calder. The system was also adopted at the military camps at Aldershot, Sheerness and Woolwich.[47] When these closets were 'well managed', that is, thoroughly lined and emptied regularly, they were clean and inoffensive, but in many cases sanitary inspectors found the solid excreta was not kept dry: then they were no better than unprepared tubs.[48] Bucket closets, typically supplied with a wide-topped galvanised iron bucket became common in many rural parts of Britain in the late nineteenth century, but often, it would appear, without the aid of ash, earth or any other lining. Writing of Somerset in 1915, William Savage reported, 'Bucket closets are now fairly common; they are intended to be used as earth closets, but in my experience it is rare to find earth used'.[49]

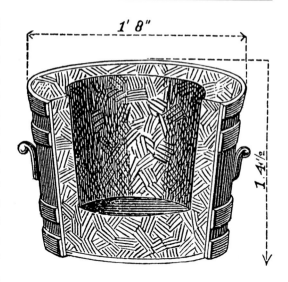

The Goux tub, as used in Halifax in the 1880s, containing a lining of various absorbent materials, 3 or 4 in thick at the base and 3 in at the sides. In wool towns like Halifax, the urine was often collected separately for use in local mills to remove the grease naturally occurring in wool.

In some towns, the pail system survived into the early twentieth century, with the collection of pails maintained by the local authority, although by then it was regarded as most unsatisfactory.[50] The operation of dry closets in towns – especially if earth was to be used – could present major practical difficulties. In 1872, the influential agricultural scientist, Dr Augustus Voelcker (1822–84), argued that in towns the water-closet plan provided the quickest, cheapest and healthiest way of disposing of waste. Carting the bulky dry waste to the countryside for use as manure was expensive and, in his opinion, hardly cost-effective. Some five-sixths of the fertilising value of the manure was found in the urine, but this was lost to the dry soil, much of which, Voelcker pointed out, consisted of 'comparatively useless common earth'.[51] He conducted his own tests – on used earth from Wakefield prison – and discovered its nitrogen content was not particularly high, even when the earth had been used repeatedly.[52] While not doubting the disinfecting powers of fresh garden soil, Voelcker was forced to conclude that the value of the used earth as a fertiliser was not as great as enthusiastic supporters of earth closets claimed. Thus, the general use of the dry system in towns made little more economic sense than using liquid sewage as manure.

Voelcker's analysis was confined to earth and not ash closets, but ultimately, the fate of dry conservancy systems was determined not by practicalities or economics, but by people's sensitivities. In the rapidly expanding industrial towns of the north, the dry closet offered a cheap and simple solution to a problem that was expanding in direct proportion to the increase in population. In the countryside Moule's earth closet represented an enormous advance on the midden. But the simple fact is, many educated and influential people found the dry closet – in any form – revolting. Dr Angus Smith, who heaped praised on the water-carriage system in 1863, roundly condemned the attempts current at the time to develop methods of removing sewage in a dry state. For him it was 'not only the oldest, but the most objectionable of methods', which would represent a 'return to a primitive state of filth and discomfort'.[53] Smith was almost certainly voicing the majority opinion of the Victorian urban middle classes, for whom the water closet and bath tub were established as necessaries of civilised life. The dry closet was the antithesis of the modern, clean and comfortable world they wished to create. So ultimately, the impassioned arguments of Henry Moule, the ingenuity of J. Conyers Morrell and others, the exemplary organisation to be found in Rochdale and elsewhere was less important than the opinions expressed by Dr Angus Smith and clearly shared by many. In 1871 George Nelms, carpenter and builder of Woodstock, optimistically addressed his advertisement for his earth closet to 'the nobility, gentry and clergy'. Members of the nobility might have installed them in the homes of their tenants – like Lord Rothschild – but it is doubtful if few, themselves, sat on one. And as a clergyman, Moule was probably untypical in preferring an EC to a WC.[54] Moule described the water-carriage system as the 'struggling, halting rival' to the earth system.[55] But this was misplaced optimism; the water-carriage system finally won the day.

Nevertheless, Moule's earth closet and its basic cousin, the bucket, survived in the countryside until well into the twentieth century. Although Dr Voelcker had advocated the wet system, or water-closet plan, for large towns, he was, nevertheless, convinced that the dry or earth-closet plan was preferable to the adoption of sewage arrangements in villages or suburban districts 'inhabited by people in a humble position in life'.[56] In the countryside and in isolated establishments such as workhouses and prisons, disposing of the waste presented few difficulties and as expensive wet-sewage systems were rarely in place, there really was little choice. It was common in isolated homes for householders to dig a trench themselves to dispose of the contents of the buckets, although some rural district councils continued to collect the pails on a weekly basis until the 1960s.[57] With demand sustained by rural communities, designs for dry closets featured in many building and domestic manuals into the 1930s, while Moule's earth closet remained on sale in the mid-1930s. Sales of the galvanised iron buckets lasted longer – they appear in ironmongers' catalogues of the 1950s.[58] A modern bucket closet appeared in 1924 when E.L. Jackson introduced the 'Elsan' chemical toilet which used formaldehyde to kill bacteria in the waste. But generally, it was the older kind of pail closet – still to be found, like the old midden, in cottage gardens – that variously shocked, amused and fascinated visitors to the countryside throughout the twentieth century. These were not, of course, the privies known to the Saxons, the Vikings in York and earlier societies, but were the survivors of a serious attempt by progressive Victorian sanitarians to improve closets without expending vast capital sums on sewage projects only to pollute rivers and coasts.

CHAPTER FOUR

Cleanliness and Godliness

Victorian attitudes to bathing and various kinds of baths

'Cleanliness has been said to be akin to godliness,' said J. Hogg in *London As It Is*, a fascinating collection of observations and facts about the capital and its inhabitants published in 1837.[1] The Revd Charles Kingsley made the same connection when he wrote his children's story, *The Water Babies*, published in 1863. Tom, the chimney sweep's boy, had never washed himself and had never heard of God or said his prayers. And when, by chance, he saw his reflection in a mirror for the first time and found that he was dirty, he burst into tears with shame and anger. Tom was unable to wash himself as there was no water in the court where he lived.[2] Hogg also

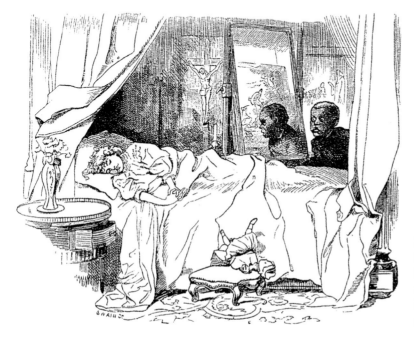

In Charles Kingsley's *The Water Babies* of 1863, Tom turns from his own reflection in the mirror to contemplate the beautiful girl sleeping under a crucifix in her white bedroom.

identified the shortage of water as a major obstacle to the health, comfort and cleanliness of London's population.

By the time *The Water Babies* appeared, regular washing and bathing was an established part of everyday life for many of the middle and upper classes. But it had not always been so. Writing in 1844, Thomas Webster said there had long been a prejudice against bathing in England.[3] For Samuel Pepys, the fact that his wife took a bath in 1665 was worthy of note in his diary, although he doubted if the occasion would be repeated. 'She now pretends,' he wrote dubiously, 'to a resolution of being hereafter very clean. How long it will hold I can guess.'[4] But taking a bath did not necessarily have much to do with keeping clean. In the eighteenth century bathing in public at a spa became fashionable: the ill – or those who thought they were ill – were drawn to the waters for their curative powers. Bathing in the sea also became popular in the eighteenth century as a means of promoting good health, but few people bathed at home to keep themselves clean.

Baths, therefore, were not common in the eighteenth century. They were installed as expensive fixtures of tile or marble in some aristocratic homes, but even at this social level they were far from common. Celia Fiennes saw a bathroom on her travels at Chatsworth in 1697. Wimpole Hall in Cambridgeshire contains a large sunken bath added by Sir John Soane around 1792 for the 3rd Earl of Hardwicke, and a similar example was installed in the basement of 7 Great George Street, Bristol, built in about 1790 for John Pinney, a wealthy Bristol sugar merchant. A smaller and later example also survives in a house in Sydney Place, Bath, an imposing terrace completed in about 1811, which was home to some of the wealthiest and fashionable in Bath at the time. This plain rectangular bath, 80 in long and 29 in wide is located at the rear of the upper-ground floor; steps in the bath lead down to a maximum depth of about 6 ft. A rare glimpse of a bath lower down the social scale survives in an inventory of 1725: the garret of a Shropshire inn contained 'one old bathing tub'.[5] Like bathing in public, a domestic bath was often taken as a cure or at least as a means of easing the symptoms of illness. In Bristol, John Pinney – who was something of a hypochondriac – wrote in October 1761, 'I now subscribe to a cold bath & goes in every morning which I finds to be of great service to me.'[6] The French revolutionary, Jean Paul Marat (1744–93) was famously murdered in a full length or slipper bath by Charlotte Corday while easing the symptoms of his eczema. In 1833, the encyclopaedist, J.C. Loudon (1783–1843) remarked on the 'many different kinds of baths available and that he had occasion to try several of them . . . in consequence of ill health at various periods during the past forty years'.[7]

James Jennings's *Family Cyclopaedia*, published in 1821, and clearly aimed at a literate middle-class audience was typical in drawing a distinction between personal cleanliness and bathing.[8] In this A to Z of domestic matters the two subjects were given separate entries. 'Personal cleanliness of the person and of the dress,' he acknowledged, 'is not only becoming in our intercourse with society, but is absolutely necessary if we desire that invaluable blessing good health.' He recommended frequent washing of the face, hands and feet and occasionally of the whole body adding that, 'there is no objection to the use of soap'.[9] Jennings advised his readers that the linen or cotton worn next to the skin should be changed at least twice a week and stockings oftener. Jennings briefly acknowledged that a bath could be used for washing and cleaning – in which case it was a 'soap bath' – but most of his lengthy discussion on the subject of bathing was related to health. Hands and face were usually washed with the aid of a washstand equipped with a basin and a few jugs. The washstand had appeared before the end of the eighteenth century, and throughout the nineteenth century was virtually a standard article of bedroom furniture among the better-off. In *The Water Babies* when Tom mistakenly emerges from a chimney into the bedroom of a beautiful (and very clean) little girl at Harthover House, he was puzzled to find a washing stand with ewers and basins, soap, brushes and towels. There was also a bath filled with clean water – 'what a heap of things all for washing!'

The use of baths appears to have increased in the early decades of the nineteenth century. Whatever the assumed benefits of taking a bath, more information on the subject became available in the 1820s and 1830s as an expanding number of medical dictionaries and manuals of domestic economy were published. Bathing was also brought to a wider audience through printed advertising. From the early 1800s, advertisements for baths, along with all kinds of other household goods, were increasingly inserted in trade directories, newspapers and journals by furnishing ironmongers. Specialist bath manufacturers had appeared by the 1830s: Ewart and Sons of the New Road, Euston, London, who were to become leading makers of baths, were established in 1834. Rippon and Burton of Oxford Street, London, advertised their range of baths in the third instalment of Charles Dickens's *The Life and Adventures of Nicholas Nickleby*, published by Chapman and Hall in July 1838. Prices started at 6s – well within the reach of the middle-class reader of popular novels.

Having the sufficient means to purchase a bath, of course, was fundamental, but being middle class was never entirely a matter of income or occupation. The Victorian middle classes were united by a strong sense of respectability, sobriety and good manners. The home was the centre of their existence. They were intensely house-proud and particularly concerned with the degree of comfort and luxury in their homes. The trials and tribulations of the middle-class family trying to improve their lot was lampooned in *Punch* during the 1840s and 1850s. The hapless Mr Briggs is shown struggling with smoky chimneys, the Fogies try to grapple with the complexities of a 'new-fangled' oil lamp and in 1850 'paterfamilias' brandishes a scrubbing brush of frightening proportions as his tearful children prepare for a shower bath. Creating a routine of regular bathtime for the family was an expression of middle-class values: it was an effective way of promoting good health, cleanliness – and therefore respectability – and perhaps even, if the water was cold, character training.

'Hot baths are by no means a class of agents to be trifled with, and in medical cases where there is time to obtain it, regular advice should be had recourse to before using them.' J.H. Walsh, 1857.

Promoting good health remained fundamental to ideas on bathing. This was no simple matter: bathing took many forms and so the effects on the body varied according to the type of bath. Jennings drew a basic distinction between the 'general' bath where total immersion – or plunging – took place and the 'partial' where water was thrown on to the body as in a shower bath. In his *Domestic Encyclopaedia* of 1844, Thomas Webster said baths could be seen as either curative (the 'therapeutic' bath) or as preventative (the 'hygeian' bath), that is, a bath which preserved good health.[10] Baths were also subdivided according to the temperature of the water. A cold bath, according to Webster, 'strengthens the digestive organs' and was best taken in the mornings, and a cold shower, rather than a plunge was the most effective method of cold bathing. 'Its effects', he wrote, 'are more speedy and extend more to the internal organs than those of the common bath.'[11] Curiously, no distinction was made between outdoor bathing in rivers, ponds and the sea and having a bath at home. Thus, a cold bath could equally be taken in a river. For Jennings, only the timing was different: he preferred the afternoons or 'from one to two hours before sunset' for river bathing. The shock suffered from sudden contact with cold water was considered beneficial in cases of fever and Jennings claimed that the cold bath had cured cases of tetanus, epilepsy, rabies – and even insanity. Cold baths were not for the timid. They had to be approached with boldness and resolution so that the cold water should come into contact at once with the entire body. The nineteenth-century cold bath was clearly a masculine pursuit, an ideal way to train the characters of young gentlemen. Morning cold baths became part of the regime in many public schools. The warm or tepid bath, in contrast, was recommended for 'delicate females' and infants. J.H. Walsh summarised the benefits of warm baths in his domestic manual of 1857: 'warm baths,' he wrote, 'soothe the general nervous system and are of great use in spasms of any kind as well as in convulsions of young children', Much of the detail concerning the health benefits and effects on the body of different types of bath varied according to the author, but on one important matter they were in total agreement: hot baths were potentially dangerous. 'Hot baths,' said Walsh, 'are by no means a class of agents to be trifled with, and in medical cases where there is time to obtain it, regular advice should be had recourse to before using them.'[12] The bather, therefore, was the patient: a medical dictionary a more likely bath accessory than a bar of soap.

But was it? While early Victorian writers remained preoccupied with the medical functions of bathing, its popularity – particularly among the literate middle classes – coincided with the rise of the public health movement, which raised awareness of the connection between disease and dirt. By the early nineteenth century, there was a growing realisation that people who kept themselves clean were more likely to enjoy good health. James Jennings had pointed this out in 1821. Moreover, clean people found other clean people socially respectable – and dirty people less so, even offensive. Cleanliness, like good manners became an indicator of respectability while dirt and squalor were seen as threats to moral as well as physical health. Describing the filthy and insanitary state of houses in Christmas Street, Bristol in 1843, Dr Budd said, 'people living among [such conditions] necessarily become coarse, filthy and brutalised'.[13] To be clean was to be decent, and so cleanliness and godliness became axiomatic of Victorian middle-class life. So many people who added bathing to their domestic routine in the nineteenth century were probably more concerned with keeping themselves clean than with treating convulsions, rabies or insanity. Over time the importance of high standards of personal hygiene gained wider currency. *Cassell's Household Guide* of 1869 hardly mentioned the medical dimension of bathing and instead wrote of the importance of the 'Saturday night wash'.[14] Two decades earlier Webster had hoped the importance of bathing would extend to all, particularly the working classes. But the working classes, themselves, probably remained largely oblivious to the benefits of bathing. In the mid-nineteenth century water was still scarce; filling a bath was usually a job for servants and taking a bath, therefore, largely confined to the servant-owning middle and upper classes.

'Hot baths should be only taken as a rule as a cleansing operation; in fact, for the Saturday night's wash so to speak.'
Cassell's Household Guide *c.* 1869.

With so many ideas current about the nature of bathing it is hardly surprising that there was an extraordinary variety of baths in use

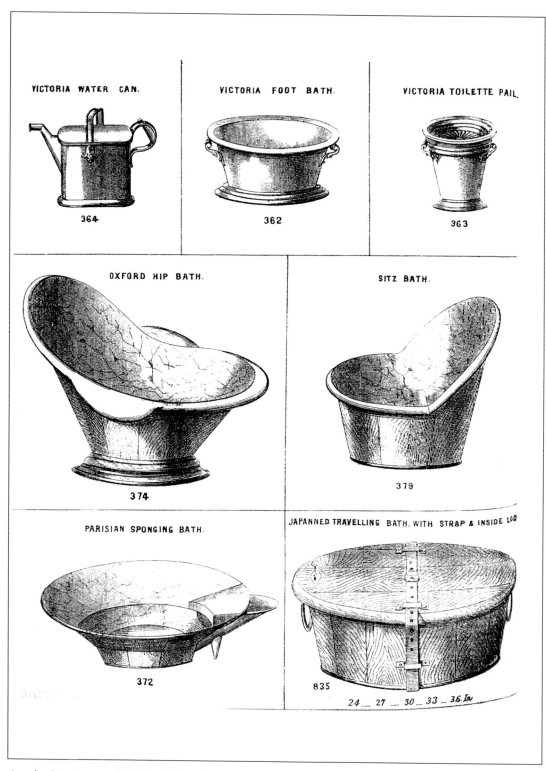

A trade advertisement of 1868 for baths and toilet-ware made by Edward Perry, Wolverhampton. West Midland tinplate manufacturers were important makers of portable baths and toilet-ware at this time. (*Rural History Centre*)

during the nineteenth century. Unlike the large, deep-water baths found in some large Georgian houses, the typical early and mid-nineteenth-century bath was small and portable. They were easier to fill – and cheaper to buy – although it was not so easy to experience total immersion. Wooden tubs may have been used but most middle-class families would have aspired to own a bath made for the purpose by furnishing ironmongers and metal workers out of tinned sheet iron. Baths were also made of copper, but they were more expensive. Portable baths came in a wide range of shapes and sizes. Probably the most popular type was the hip bath in which the bather's hips were immersed in a round or oval basin tapering downwards with a base which tapered outwards for stability and a high rounded back. The lower legs and arms extended somewhat uncomfortably outside the bath, although many had arm rests on the rim. Sitz baths were similar but had a seat in the back and no flared base. In 1863, Henry Loveridge and Co. of Wolverhampton, then one of the largest manufacturers of japanned (stove varnished) ware in the Midlands, advertised a hip bath with a hollow inner rim designed to prevent the water slopping over the side, thus 'preserving the carpet and room from wetting and injury'.[15] In 1873, another Wolverhampton

'Washing Trotters', the original title of this engraving by Thomas Rowlandson (1756–1827) of a couple washing their feet in a wooden-staved tub, published by Hixon, Strand, London, 1800. (*British Museum*)

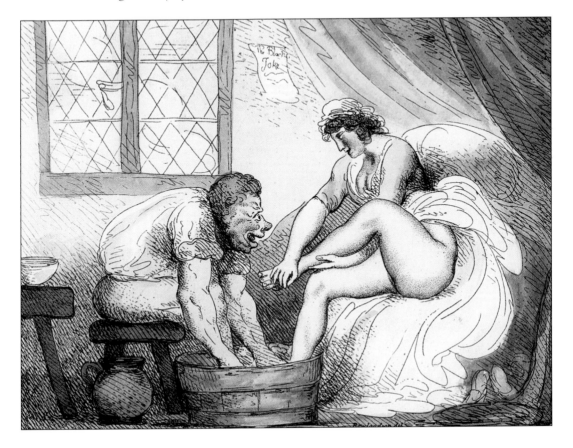

maker, Jones Brothers, advertised a hip bath shaped like a drawing-room armchair.[16]

Then there were foot baths and leg baths. Thomas Rowlandson (1756–1827) shows a couple washing their feet in a wooden coopered tub in a drawing of 1800. They were also made in tinplate and earthenware and consisted of tub-shaped bowls with handles at the sides; knee-high versions resembling large boots were called leg baths.[17] Earthenware foot baths had appeared by the 1790s, and like other items of toilet-ware were made with attractive underglaze decoration. A book of *Cookery and Domestic Economy* for 'young housewives in the middle ranks of society', written by 'the Mistress of a Family' in 1845, provided advice on the best type of foot baths. 'Few houses possess the convenience of baths, but every one may command the use of small movable vessels for the feet or for infants. The best kind of foot and leg bath is a deep wooden pail; those of earthenware are exceedingly liable to break, and besides are very expensive.'[18]

Full-length baths were also available by the early nineteenth century, but it is doubtful if they were ever as widely used as the smaller types. They went by a variety of names: slipper baths, lounge baths and ladies' baths and could be double-ended, that is, parallel-sided with matching curved ends, or tapered. Some slipper baths were fully enclosed, resembling giant slippers or boots of iron – this is the type of bath in which the murdered Marat is sometimes shown in prints. They were made in Britain during the first half of the nineteenth century: a surviving example by Bishop, ironmongers in Bath between about 1805 and 1854, consists of some twenty-five individual pieces of sheet metal riveted together. It originally

'The hip or sitz bath is a valuable remedy either hot or cold . . . when hot it allays spasm or irritation about the bladder or lower bowels or any of the organs within the pelvis.'
J.H. Walsh, 1857.

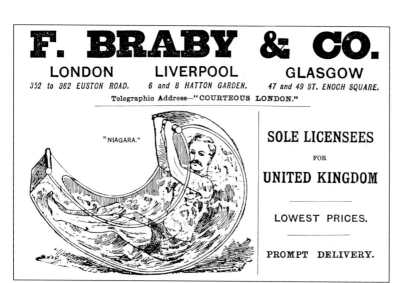

F. BRABY & CO.

LONDON   LIVERPOOL   GLASGOW
352 to 362 EUSTON ROAD.   6 and 8 HATTON GARDEN.   47 and 49 ST. ENOCH SQUARE.
Telegraphic Address—"COURTEOUS LONDON."

"NIAGARA."

SOLE LICENSEES
FOR
UNITED KINGDOM

LOWEST PRICES.

PROMPT DELIVERY.

The 'Niagara' rocking bath made by F. Braby and Co., patented by F.A. Thyss in 1891. The curved bottom enabled the bather to rock the bath and the ends and sides were bent inwards to prevent splashing. *The Ironmonger,* 9 July 1892. (*Rural History Centre*)

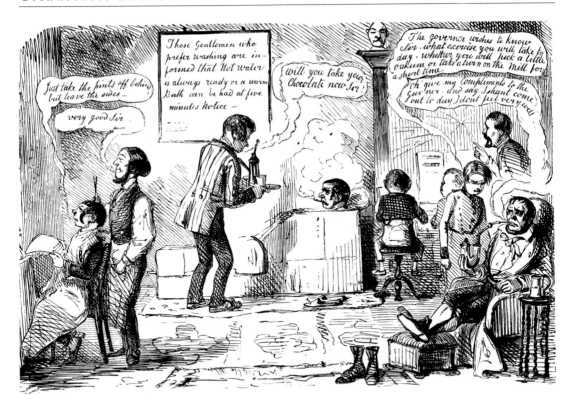

contained a brass drain cock in the 'toe' for releasing the used water.[19]

Jennings's 'partial bath' where water was thrown against the body was principally of two kinds: the sponge and the shower bath. By using a sponge bath contact with water could be kept to an absolute minimum. The bath was nothing more than a shallow, tinplate iron bowl about 3 ft wide with a spout for pouring off the used water. Some were even provided with a central platform that served as a small island to keep the feet above the water. Standing in the shallow bowl – perhaps with dry feet – the bather bent down and filled a sponge with water which was then squeezed out, first over the back and then the chest. Sponging like this could even be done under a loose dressing gown. 'The medical profession is unanimous', claimed the London manufacturers, Groom and Co., advertising their sponge bath in 1882, 'in condemning the practice of standing in cold water while taking a bath because doing so drives the blood to the head.'[20] They provided a platform along one side of their sponge bath so that the bather could avoid the upward rush of blood. The same year, Jones Brothers and Co. of Wolverhampton introduced their 'Elysian' bath supplied with a movable wooden seat, which placed in the centre of the bath served as a foot stand or placed across the spout could be used as seat when washing the feet.[21] The sponge bath was

This cartoon by John Leech originally appeared in *Punch* with the caption, 'How to make culprits more comfortable: or, hints on prison discipline'. A prisoner relaxes in an enclosed slipper bath smoking a cigar as a warder arrives with his chocolate. *Punch*, 1849.

inexpensive, easy to store (under the bed) and like the hip bath appears to have been widely used. Recalling her time as a post-office assistant in a north Oxfordshire village in the 1890s, Flora Thompson described the, 'large, shallow saucer shaped bath' used by Miss Lane, the postmistress for her 'canary dip' – a bath taken weekly in a 'few inches of warm rain water well laced with eau de cologne'. Flora herself, however, preferred using a hip bath in which she could at least have a 'good hot soak'.[22]

Shower baths had appeared by about 1810.[23] Jennings refers to them in 1821 and the first patent for one taken out by John Benham, a leading London furnishing ironmonger, in 1830, describes improvements, 'applicable . . . to the common shower bath'. The typical shower bath had an overhead cistern usually

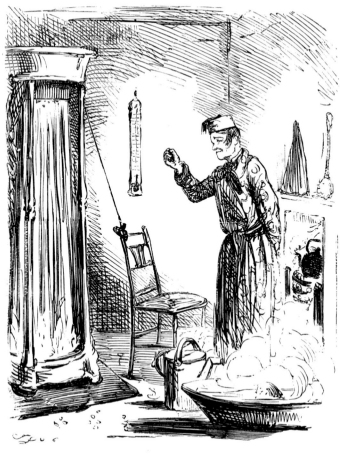

supported by four uprights fixed to a simple round bowl: the London brass founders, John Warner and Sons, called this a 'pillar' shower bath in their 1856 catalogue.[24] The cistern was also combined with hip baths, and Walsh, in 1857, shows a shower cistern fixed above a full-length bath. The cistern had to be filled by hand – as illustrated in a famous cartoon by John Leech which appeared in *Punch* in 1850 – or they were fitted with a pump which the user could work to raise the water from the bath to the cistern. To release the shower water the bather stepped into the tub, closed the curtain, which was usually suspended from a rail attached to the base of the cistern, and then pulled a string which opened a valve allowing water to pass through the perforated base of the cistern. They were not cheap: in the late 1830s a shower bath cost £4, although in 1844 Webster did admit that a large tin colander would do the job, providing an attendant was present on a pair of steps to pour in the water. Benham's patent of 1830 claimed the addition of perforated horizontal pipes to the shower bath as his invention. Upon turning a water cock the user was subjected to the pleasant sensation of

The original caption of this *Punch* cartoon by John Leech was, 'Quite a new sensation for the luxurious, on cold mornings, Use hot water and look at your shower bath!' The sponge bath (with a sponge in place) has just been filled with steaming hot water from the can, while a conical shower cap and scrubbing brush sit unused on the mantlepiece. A thermometer on the wall suggests that the room is rather chilly in spite of the blazing fire. *Punch*, 1849.

horizontal jets of water in addition to the usual downward shower. Unfortunately, the pleasant sensation was of short duration and limited strength. The pressure of the shower – and spray, if fitted – was governed by the height of the cistern above the bath and the quantity of water it held. Once the water was released the power of the spray rapidly diminished and soon dwindled to a trickle as the cistern emptied. At best a shower would last only a few minutes. Their effectiveness depended upon a constant supply of water, and when this eventually became widely available in the later nineteenth century, combined shower and spray baths became fashionable among the well-to-do.

Bathing usually involved contact – if not immersion in water – but not always. The steam or vapour bath, in which the medium was steam, received serious attention. They were based on bathing practices from Russia and Turkey. Steam was produced from water in a vessel heated by a small stove and conveyed by pipes to the bather seated on a chair enclosed in a wagon-like frame of cane, whalebone or wood and covered in blankets. Alternatively the steam could be fed to a cabinet of some sort in which the bather could sit. The steam bath, according to Webster, was particularly 'efficacious for gout and rheumatism'. William Flavel, an iron founder and kitchen-range manufacturer in Leamington Spa, fabricated a vapour bath for a visiting Russian nobleman, Major-General Sabloukoff and his family in 1815.[25]

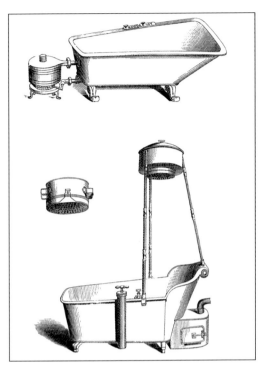

The ultimate in mid-nineteenth-century luxury: a full-length bath fitted with an overhead shower and a small solid fuel stove for heating the water. Walsh's *Manual of Domestic Economy*, 1857.

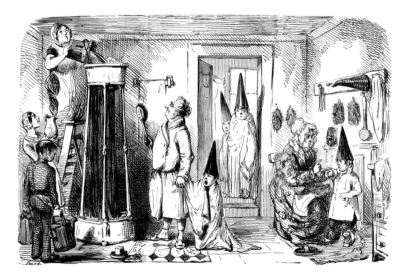

This cartoon by John Leech shows a typical mid-nineteenth-century shower bath. Bath-time is clearly a traumatic event for the young bathers made to wear oil-skin shower caps resembling a dunce's hat. The cistern takes three servants to fill using a miscellaneous collection of jugs and buckets, in addition to the typical water can carried by the youth in the foreground. Father brandishes a fierce-looking flesh brush and there appears to be a bar of soap on a dish beside the shower. *Punch*, 1850.

However, Flavel's future success was secured through their famous cooking range, the 'Leamington Kitchener' – and not vapour baths – and although several received honourable mention at the Great Exhibition in 1851 they never enjoyed the success of more conventional baths.

Varying considerably in shape, size and cost all these baths, however, had one thing in common: they were not fixtures but portable. They had no room of their own. Before the 1870s bathrooms remained the exception. The portable bath was essentially an item of domestic furniture and made to look the part with japanned exteriors decorated with bamboo patterns or given the popular oak-grained mid-brown finish. Interiors were usually white or marbled in a light colour. Portable baths could even travel with their owners and some were made to fold into specially constructed leather travelling cases. In June 1863 Henry Loveridge and Co. advertised a patent travelling hip bath in time for the commencement of the seaside

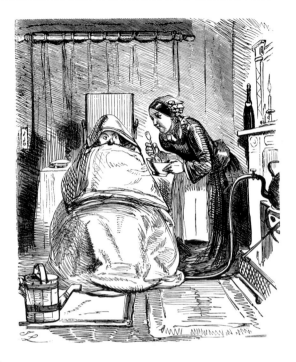

Mid-nineteenth-century domestic manuals made taking a vapour bath look so straightforward – the perfect cure for a head cold – but in this cartoon, John Leech shows just how wrong things could go! *Punch,* 1856.

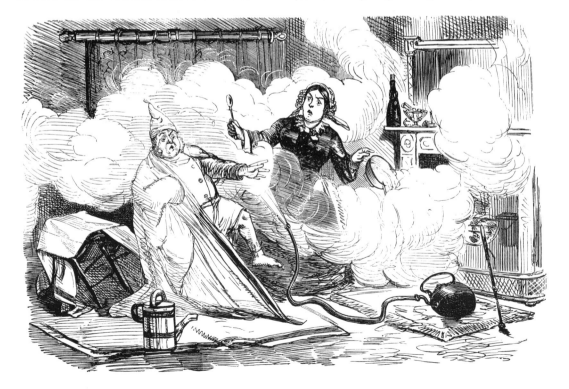

season: this had a removable lid and carrying strap enabling the bath to double as a travelling trunk.[26] As items of furniture they were an affordable purchase, at least for the growing middle classes: in the middle of the century a hip bath cost about £1 – no more than the price of some kitchen utensils. Providing the householder with ample choice was clearly an important consideration for the makers and retailers and contributed to the wide variety of baths available. Their individual identity was underlined by names: thus J.D. Clark, tinplate manufacturers of Worcester, sold 'Windsor', 'Malvern', and 'Athenian' hip baths – all with detail differences, and from the 1850s to as late as the 1920s the 'Oxford' was a popular trade name for hip baths. By the end of the nineteenth century the bath had largely become a builders' fixture: the element of choice was perhaps of less importance and most people came to accept the ubiquitous full-length rectangular bath.

Until after the 1850s the greatest practical obstacle to the use of baths at all social levels was the shortage of adequate water supplies. According to Webster, many of the best houses in the West End of London contained the service pipes of the water companies, which conducted water to the bed-chamber floors,[27] but in the 1840s, this was still exceptional. Bathrooms with a supply of water were rare before the 1870s and baths were taken in bedrooms or adjoining dressing rooms. They were filled or emptied by hand – usually by servants, and so bathtime was a major domestic event. First a good fire was lit in the room and then the bath brought out and placed in front of the hearth on large towels or a piece of oil cloth to protect the carpet from splashes. Then the hard work began. The bath was gradually filled using cans specially made for the purpose with short, squat spouts and a lid. The number of journeys depended, of course, on the size of the can and type of bath, cans large enough to hold three gallons were sometimes used and a couple of canloads this size would suffice for a hip or sponge bath. Less still would be required for a foot bath, but full-length baths took a lot of filling: even a meagre bath of 4 to 6 in of water would require 12 gallons weighing over a hundredweight, while a luxurious soak in a full bath would need at least double this quantity. In the typical, large town house, all this water had to be carried up two floors from the basement kitchen.

The bath filled, the bather was then free to soak in comfort, facing the fire, protected from draughts by a screen or covered towel horse and perhaps resting against a cushion placed on the back of the bath. Soap and a flannel or sponge were not essential accessories, but the mid-Victorian male bather probably made sure he enjoyed his bath armed with a newspaper and a cigar. Upon rising from the bath, the

'Miss Lane took what she called her "canary dip" in a large, shallow saucer shaped bath in her bedroom in a few inches of warm rain water well laced with eau de cologne.'
Flora Thompson, 1945.

bather took a warm towel from the towel horse and walked away. The dirty bath water was left for the servants to deal with. Not surprisingly, full-length baths were unpopular because of the quantity of water they required. In her *Household Organisation* of 1877, Florence Caddy acknowledged the drudgery created by bath-time: 'Men will do much for glory and vainglory,' she wrote, 'even to using cold shower baths in winter and boast of breaking the ice in them but I never yet heard of a man who took the trouble to empty his bath after using it'. She added, 'when a man likes to have his bath regularly he should think of the labour that half a dozen or more baths entail and in the evening prepare his own can of water . . . and say nothing about it'.[28] Carrying even cold water to the bath was one major practical difficulty in preparing a bath, but when the bath was to be taken warm or hot, another was heating the water.

The hot-water can was usually filled from the boiler at the side of the kitchen range. These had become a common feature of ranges from the 1780s[29] and usually had a brass cock or tap at the front to draw off the water manually. But if the range was not in use – which was more likely in summer – it was inconvenient and expensive to light the kitchen fire just to supply bath water. So baths with their own source of heat were devised. J.C. Loudon referred to portable self-heating baths in 1833, although without much enthusiasm. They came with a small coal-fired stove and boiler that was connected to the bath by flow and return pipes: these enabled the hot water to flow into the bath while colder water returned to the boiler. The smoke was carried away through a movable flue pipe that could be inserted in the bedroom chimney; but they were unsatisfactory in Loudon's view because of the time taken to heat the water. Notwithstanding this reservation, coal-fired baths were available as

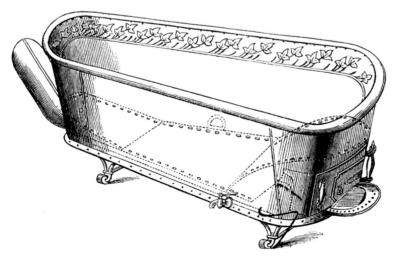

Portable hot-water bath by Chamberlain and King, Birmingham, with integral firebox and flue.
The Ironmonger, 31 August 1861. (*Rural History Centre*)

'top of the range' baths through the middle decades of the nineteenth century. In 1838, Rippon and Burton were advertising self-heating baths with a copper fireplace for £7 and claimed that the bath water could be heated safely in twenty minutes. Webster and Walsh illustrate baths in their manuals of domestic economy with separate stoves, but in 1861 Chamberlain and King of Birmingham advertised their patent hot-water bath with a firebox within the main body of the bath and a flue pipe projected from the front end.[30] Instructions for coal-fired baths emphasised the importance of filling the bath first and of extinguishing the fire before the bath was used. The bather, therefore, was spared the company of the stoker while relaxing; it also meant there was no danger of the temperature of the water rising to dangerous levels when the bath was occupied.

By the 1850s, however, self-heating baths fuelled by gas had made their debut. In 1849, Nathan Defries, a gas-stove maker in Regent Street, London, patented a means of heating water by directing jets of gas at metal plates fixed to the bottom of the bath.[31] Defries named his invention the 'Magic' heater and claimed it could heat 45 gallons of water in 6 minutes at a cost of less than *2d* of gas.[32] The bath was exhibited at the Great Exhibition in 1851 and awarded a prize medal.[33] Notwithstanding Defries's claim, gas baths usually took about 30 minutes to heat up. The effectiveness of gas for heating was then limited: its only practical application since its introduction in the early nineteenth century had been as an illuminant. The ordinary gas flame of domestic use was a lazy, low temperature, yellow flame – ideal for lighting – but less suited to heating. Nevertheless, other manufacturers introduced gas baths. In 1856, John Warner and Sons, an old established firm of brass founders in Cripplegate, London, advertised Smith's Patent gas boiler which could be fitted to one of their 5 ft 6 in 'Albert' baths. The boiler took the form of an ornate cylindrical stove with a gas burner at the bottom which could swing out for lighting, and like the coal-heated stoves was connected by flow and return pipes to the bath. The upper part of the stove held water which was heated indirectly by the boiler below and this served as a linen or towel warmer. The makers claimed grandly, 'this bath is in daily use by numbers of persons, who have already availed themselves of the opportunity of procuring so great a luxury and convenience at so moderate a price'. But Warner and Sons may not have been totally confident the idea would catch on, for they also added that the patent gas boiler could be used on its own as a greenhouse or conservatory heater with 'great economy and certainty of effect' – providing, of course, gas was laid on.

Little is known about the performance of these early gas baths: the primitive burners presumably eventually raised the bath water to the

'When a man likes to have his bath regularly . . . he should think of the labour that half a dozen or more baths entail.'
Florence Caddy, 1877.

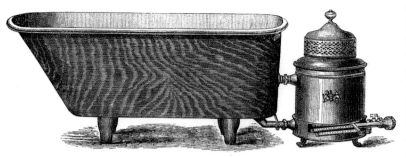

A gas bath with linen warmer
and atmospheric burner by
B. Perkins and Son, Bell Court,
Cannon Street, London. The
5 ft long bath was exhibited at
the Vienna Exhibition in 1873
where it won a prize medal.
Perkins claimed that it would
heat the water in 35 minutes;
it could be finished in
japanned green marble or oak,
white inside, with a 'bronze
green' heater and brass levers
for cold and waste; prices
ranged from £6 to £11 11s.
The Ironmonger, 1 June 1873.
(*Rural History Centre*)

required temperature, but not before they had filled the room with
soot and the smell of half-used gas. But the gas bath was to benefit
from the research of a German chemist, Robert Wilhelm Bunsen
(1811–99), who, from 1855 perfected the oxygen enriched gas
burner. By combining the gas with about 75 per cent air the flame
was transformed into a fierce, hot, blue flame. Ultimately this was to
find its greatest use in gas cookers, but for a few decades the bunsen
burner was to give impetus to the development of the gas bath. The
Victorians called it the 'atmospheric' burner, and by 1873 B. Perkins
and Son of Bell Court, Cannon Street, London, were advertising bath
stoves with atmospheric burners, which, they claimed, used only half
the gas of the usual ring burner and emitted no smell or soot 'so
objectionable in the old system'.[34] Nevertheless, they made no claim
to heat the water any quicker: their burner still took thirty-five
minutes to provide a hot bath.

The 1870s was, nevertheless, the heyday of the gas bath. Makers
such as Ewart and Sons, and George Shrewsbury of the Calda Bath
Works, Camberwell, exhibited them at provincial and international
trade fairs that had become an essential stage for manufacturers,
following the success of the Great Exhibition. Perkins's bath won a
medal at the Vienna Exhibition in 1873. The baths were given heroic
names: thus Ewart and Sons named theirs after the queen and
posthumously, Prince Albert; there was also a 'General Gordon' gas
bath, another was the 'Prince of Wales' and at the bottom end of the
market, Henry Ponder advertised a 'Cottage bath' costing £5. But
that was a lot of money for a cottager. It is doubtful if any got to use
one and the gas bath remained a middle-class luxury. Perkins's bath,
which had so impressed the Viennese jurors was fitted with an ornate
stove that could be used as a towel warmer, but from about 1870
most makers switched to placing the atmospheric burner directly
under the bath. The burner was made to swing out for lighting and
protected by a decorative fretted screen: in 1871, George Shrewsbury
even took advantage of legislation dating from 1842 to register his

*'By a proper mixture of
atmospheric air with
gas, a blue flame is
obtained which heats
faster than the ordinary
yellow flame and leaves
no sooty deposit.'*
Ewart and Sons, London,
1878.

particular design of fretwork to prevent it being copied. John Wright and Co. which emerged in the 1870s as leading makers of gas cookers and stoves in Birmingham, made gas baths with connections for supply and waste. Unlike the coal-heated bath that could still be wheeled around a bedroom on its castors, the gas bath was fixed in place by its gas pipe, its cold-water supply and the waste pipe.

The problem with the gas bath was the waiting. Ewart and Son's top model of 1878, the 'Victoria' took fifteen minutes to heat the water, but thirty minutes was more usual. In 1868, however, Benjamin Waddy Maughan, a decorative painter of Goswell Road, London, invented the geyser. Cold water entered the top of a cylindrical heating chamber and trickled down a number of spiral wires in 'finely divided films or streams' where it was heated by the rising hot gases from rows of gas jets in the base; the resulting hot water was drawn off from a tap near the bottom.[35] The waiting was almost over. In early 1874, the trade journal, *The Ironmonger*, reported that 'A very ingenious invention, the Geyser for heating water was exhibited and described (at the Inventors' Institute on 27 December 1873) by the inventor, Mr Maughan, who was present.'[36] Maughan's device was ultimately a commercial success: by 1895 Maughan's Patent Geyser Company had offices in London and Glasgow and works, the 'Geyser Factory', at Holywell Row, Finsbury, London. Soon other makers, such as Ewart and Sons and John Wright and Co., entered the field with their own versions of the geyser, all claiming that water at any temperature could be obtained instantly and that placed on a shelf at the end of the bath, the heater took up little room. In 1882 Ewart and Sons claimed that their 'Challenger' heater was 'suitable for middle-class houses in London where space is often a serious consideration'.

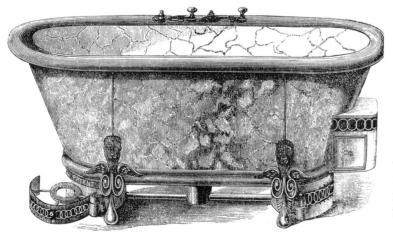

The highly ornate Victoria Patent Safety gas bath by Ewart and Sons, London. *The Ironmonger*, 19 October 1878. (*Rural History Centre*)

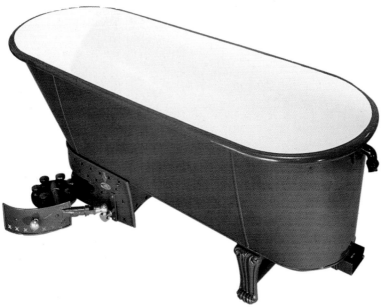

Sheet metal gas bath with swing-out burner by George Shrewsbury, London, *c.* 1871.

The geyser and its imitators were a potent weapon in the struggle of the gas-stove makers – supported by the gas companies – to break the supremacy of the coal-burning kitchen range. Gas was an attractive alternative to coal as a fuel: it was cleaner and easier to use, and in the second half of the nineteenth century the price of gas was halved. From the late 1870s the gas companies began to stage cooking demonstrations at their works to convince the public that using gas was more convenient than coal. As Ewart and Sons pointed out in their advertisement for the Challenger: 'a kitchen fire however comfortable for the occupants, becomes in summer, not only to them but also to the rest of the household, a nuisance, while it is also an extravagance both in the consumption of coal and the attention required.' They continued, 'a gas stove will do all the cooking in a clean, convenient and rapid manner and a gas stove would doubtless be oftener used if it were not for the frequent objection that it provides no constant supply of hot water'. Ewart and Sons had the answer, of course: install a Challenger geyser.[37]

Maughan had taken the name for his new heater from the Icelandic word for a gusher or rager. The name was apt: water could be delivered to the bath at scalding temperatures, sometimes in alarming fits and starts. A resident of Bath recalls the working of a geyser in the 1940s: 'at the head [of the bath] towered a dragon-like copper geyser with a gas meter below for shillings. When lit, the geyser burst into life with a deafening roar and spluttered out much steam and a little water.'[38] Using a geyser could be a worrying experience in other ways. The lighting of a geyser was often accompanied by a loud bang, and if the water supply failed or was

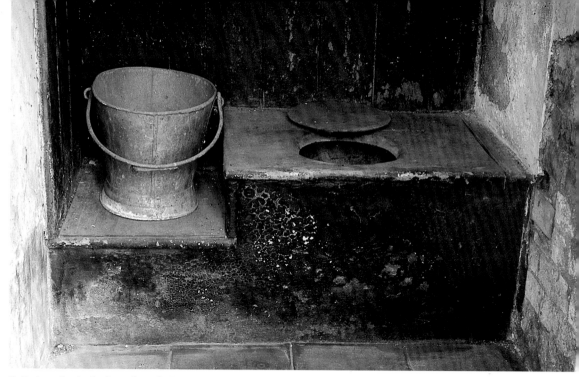

Pail closet in the back garden of a house at Tytherington, Gloucestershire, built between 1902 and 1906. The seat is hinged to remove the bucket underneath; the other bucket may have contained earth or ash to cover the excreta.

Below, left: A backyard water closet in Rosebery Terrace, Clifton, Bristol. The house was built in 1893–4 and the closet used regularly until late August 2000. It was photographed in March 2001, a few days prior to removal. The closet had a cottage pan and was set in a brick and rubble plinth under a wooden seat containing a 9-in hole. Note the vents cut in the timberwork above the doorway. *Right:* A back-garden privy at Poynings, West Sussex, last used in the 1950s. The seat had two holes, one adult sized, the other for children. It is believed the pit extended beyond the back wall, seen here; it was connected by a drain to an overflow cesspit a short distance away.

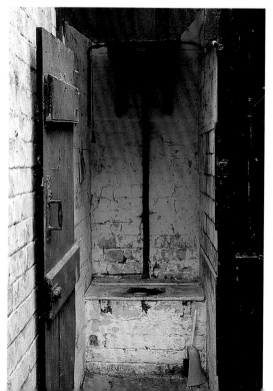

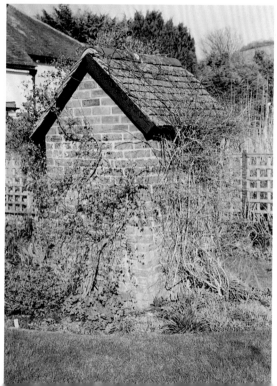

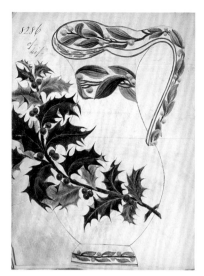

A holly design for a ewer from a Spode pattern book, *c.* 1830. (*The Spode Museum Trust*)

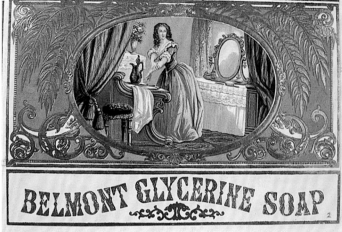

A label for 'Belmont' soap by Price's Patent Candle Co., Vauxhall, London, *c.* 1860, showing a woman using a ewer and basin to wash herself in her bedroom or dressing room.

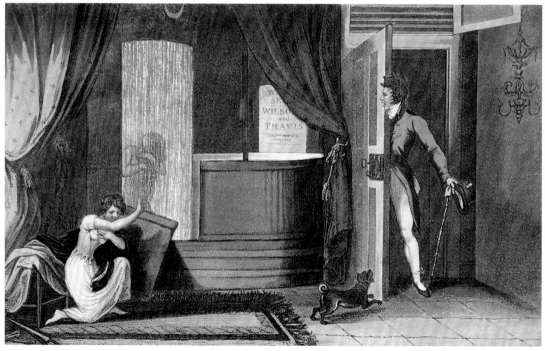

A shower bath from *Poetical Sketches of Scarborough*, 1813. The appearance of an unexpected male visitor has clearly shaken the modesty of the young woman who obviously forgot to lock the door! The shower is combined with a full-length bath. Ackermann, Strand, London, 1813. (*Mary Evans Picture Library*)

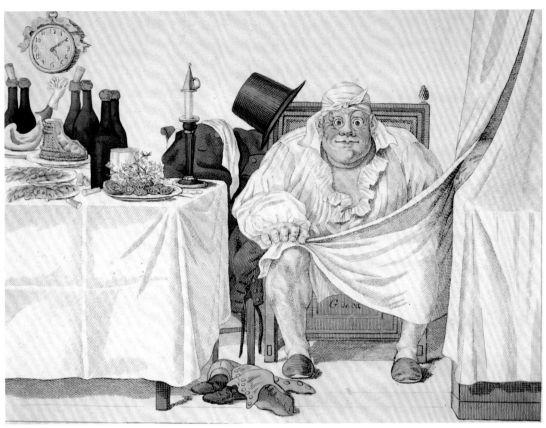

'Milord Plumpudding avec Lady Arrhée'. In this French satirical print a plump English nobleman relieves himself on a commode after tackling a hearty meal. Martinet, Paris, *c.* 1814. (*British Museum*)

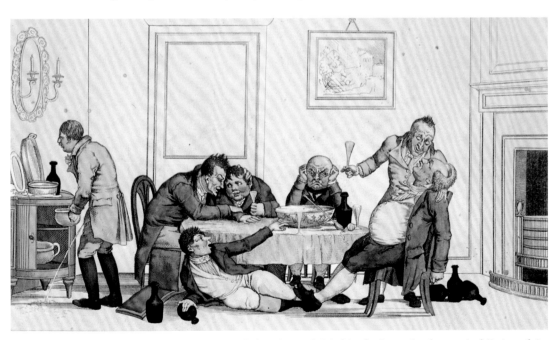

'L'Après Dinée des Anglais'. The French were appalled at the English habit of using a chamber pot in full view of the dining room. In this satirical view one of the company has left the table to use one of the two chamber pots stored in the sideboard. Although he manages to take a pot from the shelf he is so drunk he urinates on the carpet, not that his inebriated companions are in any state to notice! Martinet, Paris, *c.* 1814. (*British Museum*)

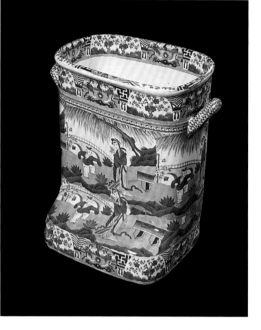
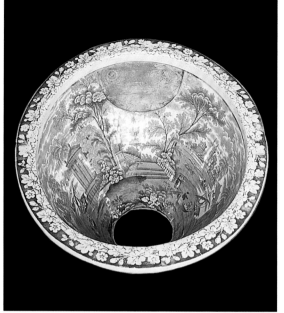
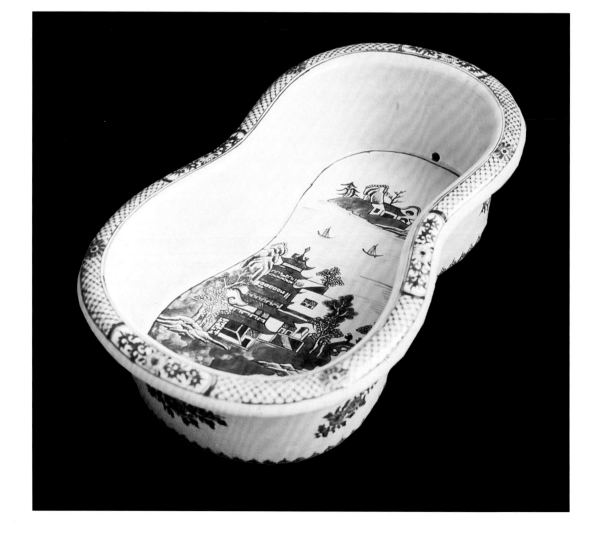

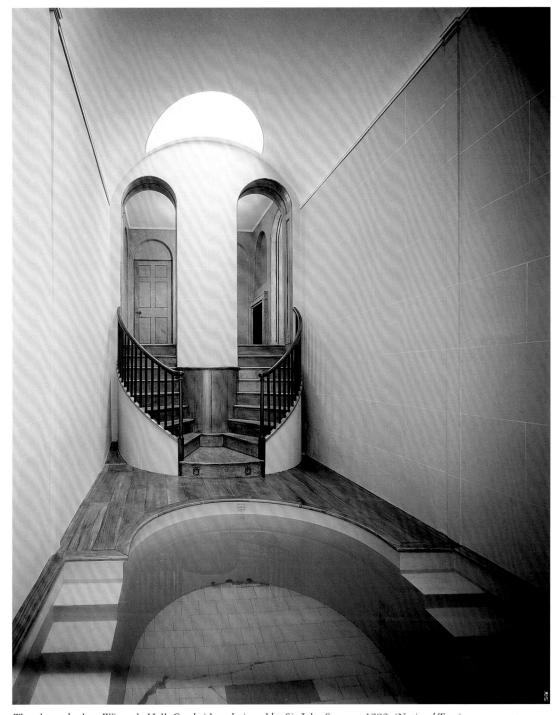

The plunge bath at Wimpole Hall, Cambridge, designed by Sir John Soane, *c.* 1792. (*National Trust*)

Opposite

Top left: Blue and white earthenware leg bath in Lange Lijsen pattern. Made by Spode, Stoke-on-Trent, *c.* 1820: height, 17¼ in. (*Spode Museum Trust*)

Top right: Blue and white earthenware basin for a pan closet, nineteenth century.

Left: Bidet in blue and white earthenware, early nineteenth century.

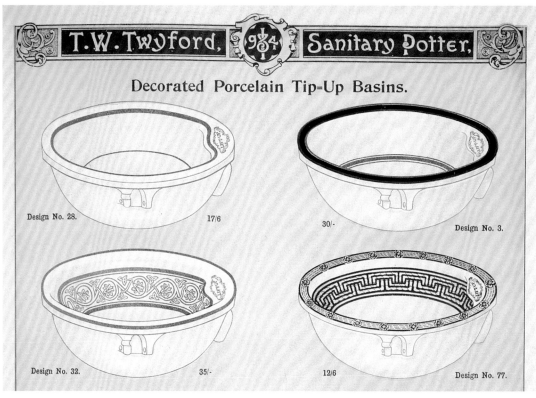

Tip-up basins in blue and gold underglaze transfer printed decoration from Twyford's 1894 catalogue. The word 'lift' is printed on the rim. (*Twyford Bathrooms*)

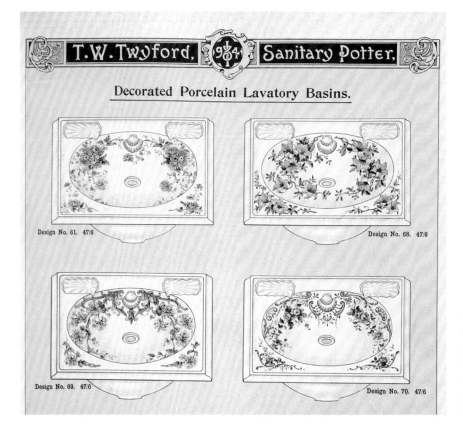

'Porcelain' lavatory basins with hand-painted and printed decoration from Twyford's 1894 catalogue. (*Twyford Bathrooms*)

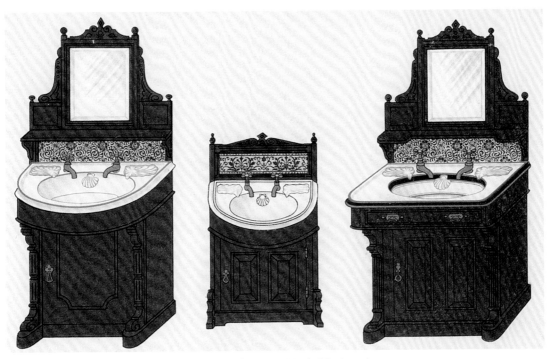

Mahogany cabinet stands from Twyford's catalogue for 1889. (*Twyford Bathrooms*)

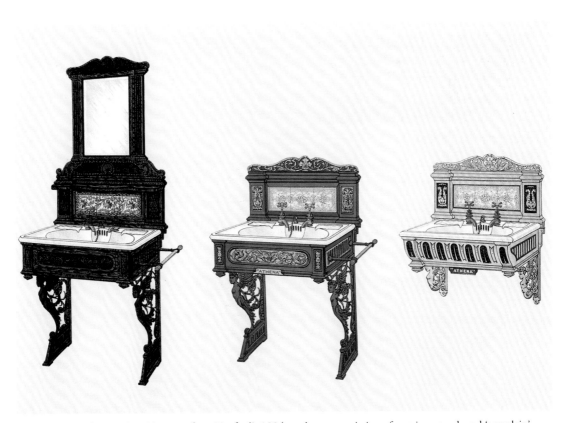

Three variants of the 'Athena' lavatory from Twyford's 1894 catalogue, consisting of cast-iron stands and 'porcelain' lavatory basins. (*Twyford Bathrooms*)

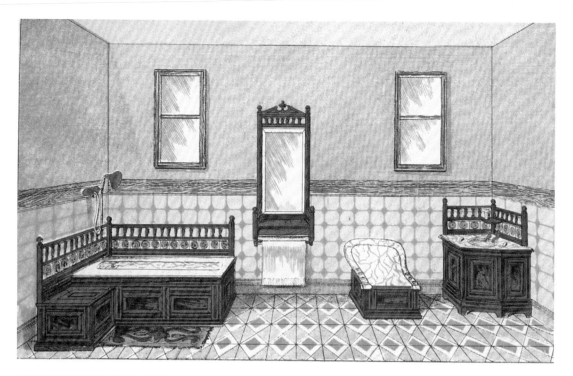

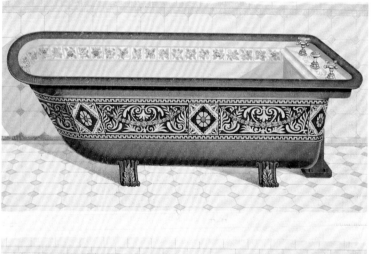

A bathroom suite of 1886 from the catalogue of T. and W. Farmiloe, London. From the left, the fittings comprised a valve closet, a full-length bath with shampoo apparatus, a mirror, sitz bath and angle lavatory washbasin in the corner. The fittings were enclosed in a choice of mahogany or walnut and the floor and walls up to a high dado level were tiled. (*Thomas Crapper and Co. Ltd*)

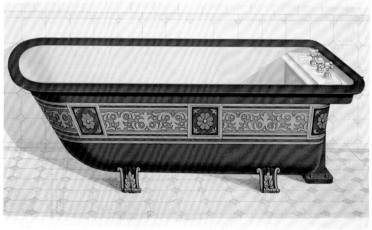

Shanks's 'Imperial' cast-iron parallel baths, *c*. 1893. By the 1890s the fashion for baths in wooden enclosures was on the wane and free-standing baths like this, decorated in metallic enamel on the outside, were becoming popular. These designs were just two of many available. The taps are set in a porcelain shelf and are of the 'noiseless and steamless' variety with the inlet near the bottom; the knob for lifting the waste outlet is in the centre. (*Mitchell Library, Glasgow*)

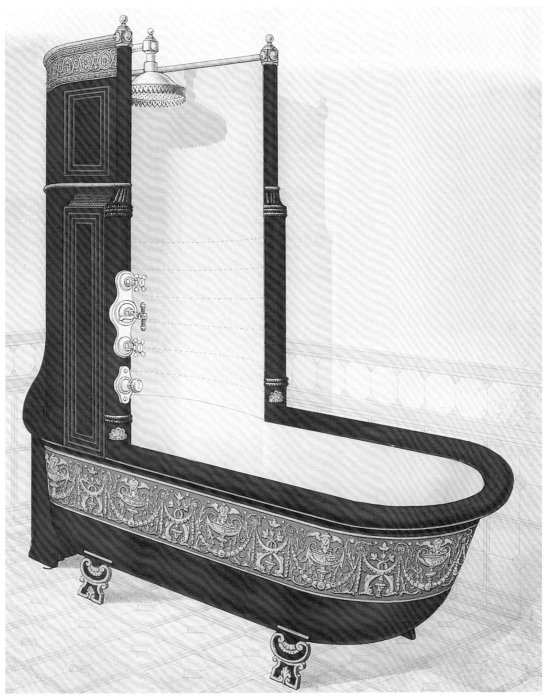

Shanks's 'Independent' spray shower and plunge bath with rolled edge and ornamental feet, *c.* 1893. This was an all-metal bath standing without a metal enclosure in keeping with the latest sanitary ideas. The drawing clearly shows the outward curve of the bath at the shower end, designed to provide a more spacious interior. The shower is nickel plated. (*Mitchell Library, Glasgow*)

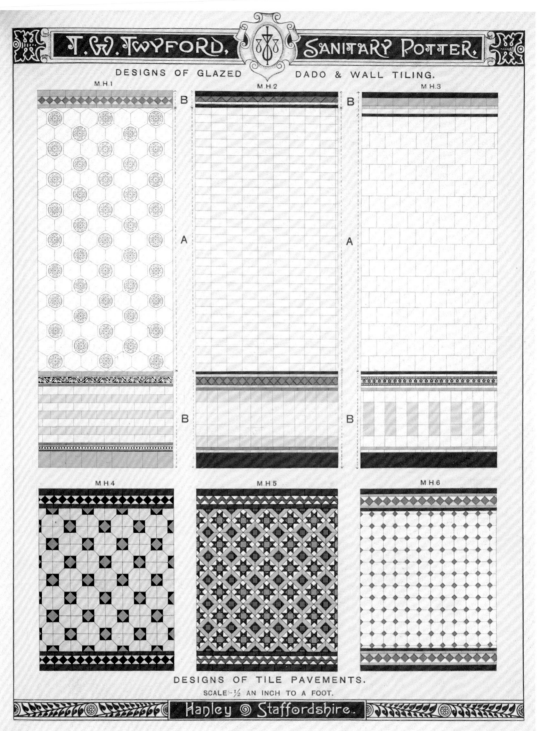

Bathroom tiles from Twyford's 1894 catalogue. (*Twyford Bathrooms*)

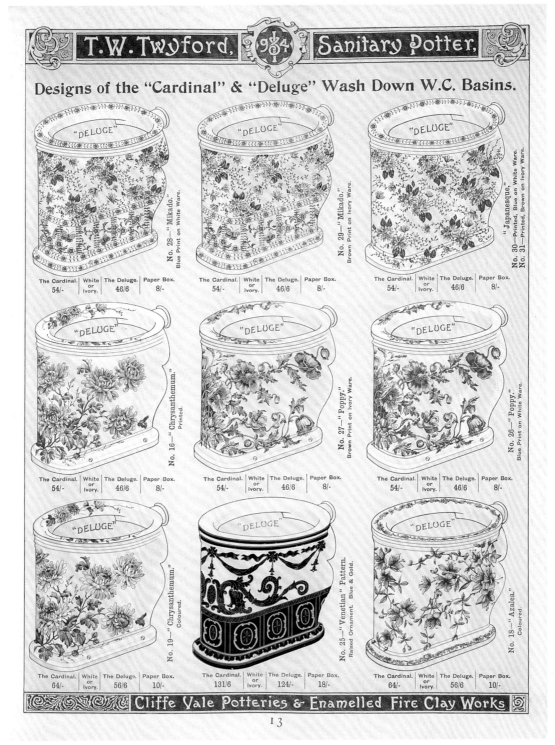

The decorated pedestal water closet reached its peak in the 1890s. Here is a page from Twyford's 1894 catalogue showing some of the designs available for the 'Cardinal' and 'Deluge' wash-down closet. (*Twyford Bathrooms*)

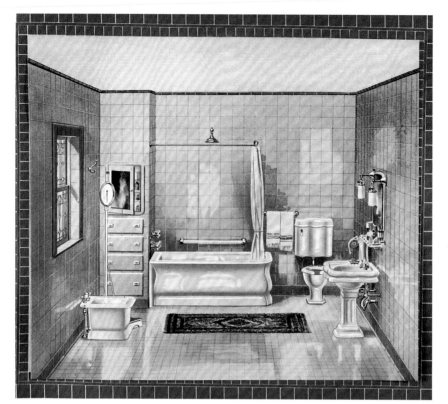

A bathroom of 1911 by the Standard Sanitary Manufacturing Co., Pittsburgh, USA. The plain white, free-standing fittings typify the uncluttered style of the hygienic early twentieth-century bathroom. Note the bathroom scales behind the foot bath. (*Mary Evans Picture Library*)

A fashionable art deco bathroom from the 1939 catalogue of Rowe Brothers of Exeter. The walls are lined with 'semi-dull' bathroom tiles with strips of 'genuine Flanders lustres', while hard dull-glazed tiles are used for the floor. The porcelain-enamelled cast-iron bath and the washbasin have the cut corners and angular styling popular in the 1930s. The lavender colour of the fittings is repeated in the skirting tiles, the rugs and even, it would appear, the towels. Note the recessed soap holder above the bath.

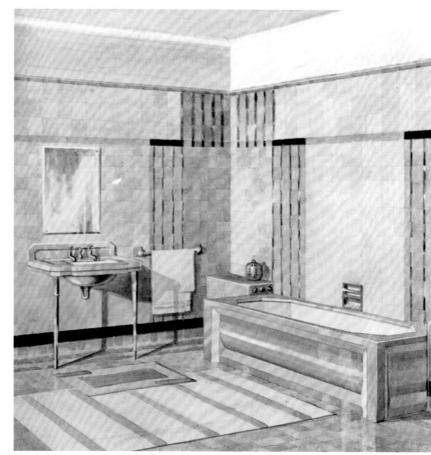

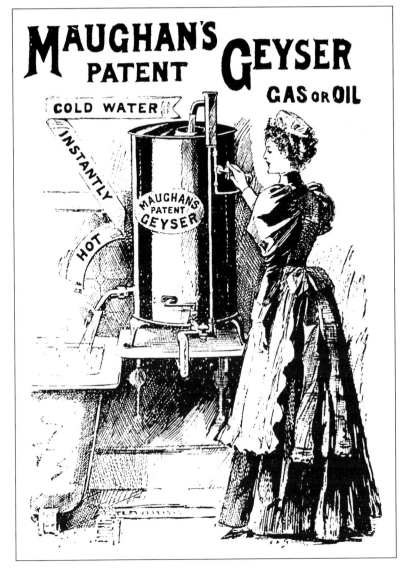

Maughan's patent geyser.
Martineau and Smith's Hardware
Trade Journal, 1895. (*Rural*
History Centre)

unintentionally turned off before turning off the gas, the geyser
would emit clouds of steam, then molten solder and finally
disintegrate. Many modifications were patented to make the geyser
safer in operation. Thus models were introduced made with a burner
carriage for lighting which interlocked the gas and water taps
ensuring a safe sequence of operations. Pilot lights were introduced
to remove the difficulty of lighting a powerful bunsen gas jet. More
seriously, these 'dragons' could kill. Geysers fitted in rooms without
adequate ventilation led to cases of bathers being asphyxiated by the
carbon monoxide they produced.

Coal heating, however, continued to rival gas as a means of
heating the bath water. In place of a stove and ungainly flue pipe

attached to the bath, manufacturers developed hot-water systems heated from the kitchen range. In 1850, Sidney Flavel, the son of William who, half a century earlier had made the vapour bath, advertised his 'Patent Kitchener' with a boiler, 'so constructed as to supply hot water to distant upper rooms, for a bath or other purpose'.[39] The boiler was placed at the back of the grate and could supply 60 or 100 gallons of hot water while the range, with its two ovens and hot plate, could be used simultaneously to bake, roast and boil or steam five or six vessels. Soon, other kitchen-range manufacturers were producing similar ranges with back boilers capable of providing piped hot water.[40] In 1857, Walsh wrote in his domestic manual, 'I believe the boiler at the back of the kitchen fire is in most houses the best method of furnishing the bath with warm water. Besides which the constant supply of hot water has now become almost a necessity in all well regulated families.'[41]

The hot-water supply was only constant, of course, when the kitchen range was lit – a disadvantage seized upon by the makers of gas heaters – but the systems that developed from the 1850s created a circulation of hot water that could be piped to anywhere in the house. This was the obvious advantage over geysers and other gas boilers that usually only heated the appliance they were attached to. The earliest circulatory arrangement adopted from the 1850s became known as the tank system.[42] It consisted of a kitchen-range boiler at the lowest point of the circulation and a hot-water storage tank at the highest, usually in the roof. Two pipes – flow and return pipes – connected the boiler and tank, creating, in effect, a 'circuit'. When the fire was lit, convection currents rose up the flow pipe while heavier, cooler water sank down the return pipe from the tank to the back boiler. Connections to draw-off pipes (and therefore, hot-water taps) were taken from the flow pipe while the hot-water tank was supplied from a cold-water cistern that was usually in the roof. As the hot water, being lighter, collected at the top of the tank it was important that the flow pipe entered near the top while the cold supply from the cistern was connected at the bottom.

There were, however, disadvantages with the tank system: opening a tap, for example, interrupted the normal circulation, and the inflowing cold water from the cistern would take the most direct route to the tap. The result was that hot water was drawn off diluted with cold. In the larger houses in which this system was usually installed, the boiler and tank were separated by several floors and so the flow pipe suffered from loss of heat; the tank in the roof also lost heat quickly. The tank system was also potentially dangerous and there were many instances of explosions. A faulty ball-cock in the supply cistern or freezing weather could stop the supply of cold

'. . . at the head of the bath towered a dragon-like copper geyser with a gas meter below for shillings. When lit, the geyser burst into life with a deafening roar and spluttered out much steam and a little water.'

A resident of Bath, 1940s.

water into the hot-water tank, but because the taps were all situated below the tank it was possible to draw off water at the lowest point until the system was nearly empty. When the small quantity in the boiler had evaporated, it would become red hot and any water returning to the empty boiler would generate steam, the pressure of which could cause an explosion. In January 1879, *The Ironmonger* reported a kitchen-boiler explosion due to the freezing-up of the supply pipes at Rock Ferry, Birkenhead, which injured two people, and another at Patricroft, Manchester which resulted in 'blowing down some of the walls of the house and severely injuring a lady and her four daughters'.[43]

By the late 1880s, the cylinder system had appeared as a safer and more efficient alternative.[44] In place of a hot-water tank in the roof, a cylinder was placed close to the kitchen range but at a slightly higher level. The hot water could be drawn off from the crown of

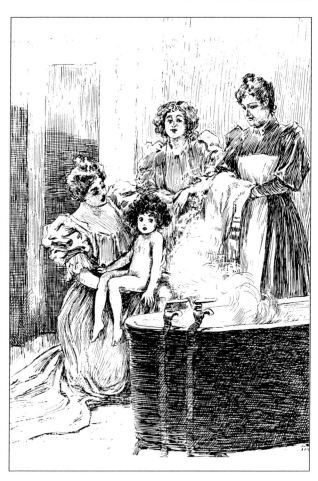

the cylinder without being mixed with cold water and another advantage was that less heat was lost as the circulating pipes were considerably shorter. The draw-off pipes were connected to the expansion pipe which extended upwards from the cylinder to above the cold-water tank in the roof and so the system could not be inadvertently emptied. Back-boiler systems were widely adopted in larger houses in the second half of the nineteenth century, particularly where mains water was laid on, which encouraged the installation of fitted baths supplied with hot and cold water. Importantly, for the servants, running hot water removed the chore of carrying it in cans from the kitchen. Moreover, the bath was now a fixture, and from the 1870s this was to give practical reality to the bathroom, the existence of which, so far, had largely been confined to theory.

In the children's story, *Two Days in the Life of Piccino*, by Frances Hodgson Burnett, the unkempt little Italian, Piccino, is lowered into a bath to be washed. But having never seen a bath before he is terrified at the prospect and thinks he might drown! By 1894, when the story appeared, fitted baths were common in middle-class homes but only thirty years earlier this scene would have been rare.

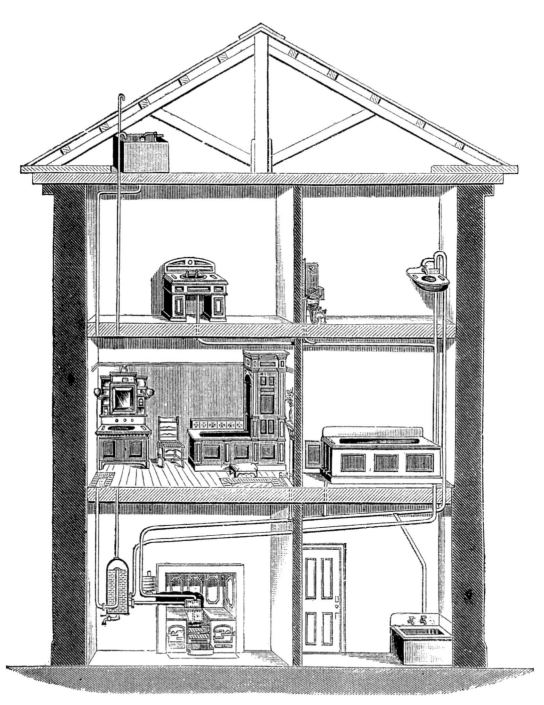

A cross-section of a house of 1889 showing a circulating hot-water system heated by a boiler at the back of the kitchen range which conducts heat to a hot-water cylinder to the left. The cold water storage tank is in the roof.

CHAPTER FIVE

Recalling Pompeii
the rise of the bathroom

The French critic and historian, Hippolyte Taine (1828–93) made several journeys through England between 1861 and 1871 and wrote of his impressions of the country and its people in his *Notes from England*, published in 1871. In this he describes, in some detail, the interior of a bedroom in a large country house. The carpeted bedroom, he observed, contained two dressing tables both with swing looking glasses. One dressing table was arranged with various utensils for washing including three jugs of different sizes, the medium-sized one being for hot water. There were also two porcelain basins, a dish for toothbrushes, two soap dishes, a water bottle with its glass and a finger glass with its own glass. 'Underneath,' wrote Taine, 'is a very low table, a sponge, another basin [and] a large shallow zinc bath for morning bathing.' And in the morning, a servant entered the room to draw the curtains and deliver 'a large can of hot water with a fluffy towel on which to place the feet'.[1]

Taine does not reveal the identity of the house, but this is not important: he was looking for the typical and what he saw was, indeed, typical of middle- and upper-class households across mid-nineteenth-century Britain. People washed – that is, took their toilet – or their bath in their bedroom or an adjacent dressing room. Taine added that the mansion had been 'arranged in the modern style'. It had three drawing rooms and had recently been refurbished at a cost of £3,000. No expense had been spared – but there was no bathroom. Bathrooms were rare also in large middle-class villas built in the 1860s, but within a few years the omission of a bathroom in affluent homes was something of an exception. By the 1890s they were even being squeezed into the floor plan of some artisan terraces, and by 1900 the bathroom was well on its way to becoming universal. In *Our Homes and How to Beautify Them*, published in 1902, H.R. Jennings wrote, 'There is a room that no self-respecting householder can do without and that is the bathroom.'[2] That this change took place within a matter of a few years was nothing short of a revolution in the domestic sphere.

Nevertheless, there was nothing new about bathrooms. The Romans were enthusiastic builders of public baths and impressive remains survive in many Roman towns across Europe, including Aqua Sulis (Bath) and Pompeii. In 1837 J. Hogg reflected, 'the magnificent baths of Diocletian [built in Rome, *c.* 305–6] remain at this day as monuments at once of the estimation in which bathing was held and of the greatness of that wonderful people'. Private baths were also found in villas and town houses of wealthy individuals, and these typically contained separate rooms for cold, warm and hot baths. Thereafter, domestic bathrooms became something of a rarity. They were largely restricted to royal circles and illustrated the wealth and status of the owner. Hampton Court, for example, begun by Cardinal Wolsey (*c.* 1473–1530) in 1515, and subsequently occupied by Henry VIII (b. 1491 r. 1509–47), contained bathrooms supplied with piped water. The French architect, Savot, included designs for bathrooms in plans for large houses published in 1624. The 'Mansion de Delices', built at Clagny by Louis XIV (b. 1638, r. 1643–1715) for his new mistress, Madame de Montespan, and completed in 1680, contained a sumptuous bathroom.[3] However, bathrooms remained rare in the eighteenth century. A Florentine bathroom is illustrated in the *Magazinno di Mobilia* in 1798, although the writer conceded that 'with us [Italians] baths are not common'.[4] The writer might well have referred to the entire continent. From the early nineteenth century, popular literature brought baths to a wider public, but so long as they remained portable utensils, often small enough to be pushed under the bed, there was little justification for a room dedicated to bathing and washing, and bathrooms remained virtually unknown before 1850.

The idea of a separate bathroom at first spread slowly. J.C. Loudon included a plan for the bathroom of a public house in his *Cottage, Farm and Villa Architecture* of 1833[5] but a decade later, the section on furnishings in Thomas Webster's comprehensive domestic encyclopaedia did not even include bathroom equipment or furnishings. Elsewhere in this book he wrote of bathing and said, 'it would be desirable that a room for bathing should be constructed in every house and though this is scarcely possible in the present condition of society yet a bath may be considered indispensable in every mansion of considerable size'.[6] J.H. Walsh referred to bathrooms briefly in his domestic manual of 1856. 'The bath', he wrote, 'may be fixed in a room specially kept for the purpose called a bathroom – or may be entirely detached.'[7] Then in 1864, the architect Robert Kerr wrote, 'no house of any pretensions will be devoid of a general bathroom'.[8]

'One may as well look for a fountain in the desert as for a bath in any of our old English houses.'

S. Stevens Hellyer, 1878.

But Kerr was, perhaps, a little ahead of many of his profession – many architects were slow at this time to make provision for bathrooms in their interior planning. It was the same with the speculative builders who were responsible for the vast majority of the middle-class villas and artisan terraces built in the nineteenth century. Most building firms were small in scale and unlikely to be at the forefront of new ideas on house layout and services. Some architects and builders of the 1870s seem to have been perhaps a little unsure about this innovation: building plans of this period occasionally show a first-floor room tentatively marked as a 'dressing room or bath-room'.

Similarly, landlords were often unwilling to incur the expense of installing bathrooms. In 1879, a surveyor writing to *The Builder* said that one of the main problems was persuading landlords to add them to existing properties: good houses, he noted, in Westbourne Terrace and Cleveland Square, London, which produced rents of between £200 and £300 per year were still without them.[9] Nevertheless, he reported that in 'recent years' it had become general to supply bathrooms to all new houses of £100 rent and above and even some houses of £50 rent – even in unfashionable London suburbs like St Peter's Park, Paddington, Shepherd's Bush and Brixton. In the third quarter of the nineteenth century, houses let at £50 a year would contain about ten rooms. A new London suburb which was to influence many later nineteenth-century suburban developments was the Bedford Park estate, developed at Chiswick between 1875 and 1881. Here red brick-detached and semi-detached houses designed in the Queen Anne style by Norman Shaw contained first-floor bathrooms and water closets.[10] The 1870s was clearly the turning point in the fortunes of the bathroom.

The practical impetus for the widespread adoption of bathrooms came from the growing popularity of the fixed bath. From the middle of the century it became increasingly common for town houses to be fitted with regular supplies of piped water, and after 1850 the English were fast becoming a nation of town dwellers. With piped water on hand connections could be made to the bath. Gas baths had just a cold supply – the burner did the heating – but many baths were fitted with hot and cold supplies: the hot water usually being heated by a boiler at the back of the range. Such baths were also fixed by their waste, or outflow, while gas baths were connected to a gas supply. As a fixture the bath created its own room, as Walsh had indicated in 1856. As a feature of palaces and large mansions, there was nothing new about the bathroom, but in the middle-class villa it was an innovation.

The small number of bathrooms built at an earlier period were usually on the ground floor – or even in basements – to lessen the

'There is a room that no self-respecting householder can do without and that is the bathroom.'
H.R. Jennings, 1902.

labour of raising the water to the bath. Furthermore, the weight of a large, sunken bath was more easily supported at ground level. But circulating water connected to lighter iron or copper baths freed the bath from the lower storeys. Piped water could be supplied to any part of the house, and as many people were already accustomed to washing or bathing in or close to their bedrooms it was but a logical step to include the bathroom in the first-floor plan along with the principal bedrooms. From the 1880s and 1890s middle-class villas were built with larger ground-floor plans so the kitchen could be located on the ground floor rather than being consigned to a gloomy basement. The larger plan also gave more space on the first floor making it easier to find space for a bathroom.

'I stepped out the bath perfectly red all over, resembling the Red Indians I had seen depicted at an East End theatre.'
Mr Pooter, 1892.

From the early nineteenth century people in larger houses had also grown used to using a water closet on the first floor, and so baths and water closet frequently came to share the one room containing all the water pipes and outlets. There was, however, some debate as to whether a bathroom should include the water closet: some believed it was more hygienic to house it in a separate room. In a paper presented at the 1879 Exhibition of Sanitary Appliances in Croydon, the sanitary reformer, William Eassie, strongly condemned the 'evil association' of bath and closet sharing the same room where 'the delivery of the bath waste is into the very foulest conduit'.[11] In 1890, Cassell's *Book of the Household* referred to 'the objectionable practice of placing a WC in the bathroom . . . common to suburban houses', calling it 'very bad and disagreeable'. The debate remained un-resolved for many decades: some of the most expensively fitted out bathrooms of the late nineteenth and early twentieth centuries included a water closet, while the typical 1930s semi-detached house usually had separate rooms for the bath and water closet.

Many tenants or occupiers (few houses were owner-occupied in the nineteenth century) wanted a bathroom. It was – as it always had been – a status symbol. 'Respectable tenants', wrote the anonymous surveyor to *The Builder* in 1879, 'will pay £5 or £10 extra rent in a moderate sized house to secure the benefit [of a hot and cold bath].' By the last decade of the nineteenth century, the adoption of the bathroom had reached to the bottom of middle-class housing. Modest villas – either semi-detached or in terraces – with from six to eight rooms were built with a small bathroom which was often situated directly over the kitchen to simplify the plumbing. Such was the home of Mr Pooter, a London clerk featured in *The Diary of A Nobody* of 1892. Pooter commuted to the City every day and lived at 'The Laurels', Brickfield Terrace, Holloway: the six-room house had a bathroom in which he took great pride, painting the bath, on one occasion, in red enamel paint – with disastrous results.[12] By the early 1900s, acquiring a bathroom became an important social indicator for the upwardly mobile artisan classes. Owning a bath demonstrated that the family cared about their cleanliness and in turn this was a statement of their respectability. Of course, there was no evidence that people washed more often once they had a bathroom.[13] Some large houses were still being built without bathrooms at the end of the nineteenth century, but now it was these which were the exceptions. By 1904 the German architect, Herman Muthesius, could write, 'England has led all the continental countries in developing the bathroom'.[14]

Muthesius also praised the modest and unpretentious interiors of English bathrooms. He found the typical English bathroom 'a simple, plain room dictated by need' in contrast to the lavish bathrooms of the well-to-do on the continent, with their high domed ceilings, opulent colour schemes and 'billowing cushions in recesses'. In reality, the picture was rather more complex, and some of the bathrooms of the wealthy in Britain were as sumptuous and luxurious as any in Europe. With few precedents or traditions to guide the householder installing a bathroom for the first time, the interior was governed by taste, budget and the space available. For the Victorian middle-class consumer, the manufacturers were not slow to draw on the past to create a traditional feel for the newest room in the house. Trade catalogues of the 1880s show bathroom interiors 'fitted in the most approved and handsome manner possible with baths supplied *en suite* with wash stands and the water closet'.[15] The idea of matching the fittings to create a unified scheme in the room followed quickly on the heels of the rise of the bathroom. And unity was achieved by enclosing the fittings in ornate wood panelling. At the International Health Exhibition in 1884 the well-known firm of sanitary engineers, George Jennings, displayed a 'very complete bath and lavatory' in the Queen Anne style with 'broken and curled pediments' over the fittings.[16]

At the same exhibition, Henry Conolly of Hampstead Road, London, exhibited a 'specimen bathroom' furnished with 'Pompeian' decorations. The ceiling was ventilated by means of a perforated cornice and the cabinetwork was, according to *The Builder*, shown *en suite* in American walnut with amboyna wood mouldings and Tuhya wood panels. The floor was covered with cork parquetry.[17] Ancient Rome and Pompeii, caught the imagination of manufacturers and consumers alike. In 1889, the Manchester firm, Morrison, Ingram and Co. advertised their 'Pompeian' spray and shower bath[18] – several manufacturers also had their 'Roman' or

'England has led all the continental countries in developing the bathroom.'
Herman Muthesius, 1904–5.

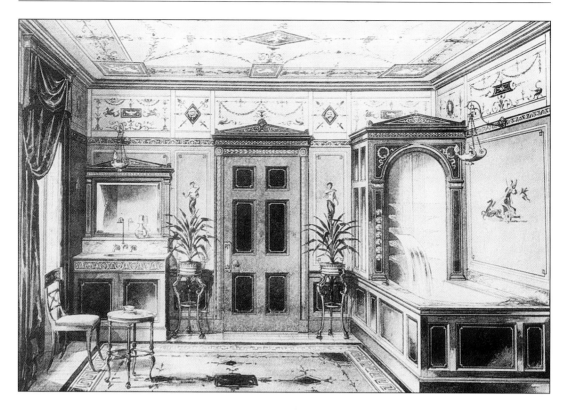

'Cleopatra' baths. The interest in classical Rome was not confined to the British. Jacob von Falke, in a work first published in Vienna in 1871 that appeared in Boston in 1878 under the title *Art in the House*, noted that the modern Frenchman took his bath in Pompeii.[19]

Von Falke was one of several writers on both sides of the Atlantic at this time who emphasised the importance of the Renaissance in forming a modern style. In 1884 Robert Kerr wrote of the enduring influence of the 'universal European Renaissance'.[20] From about 1870, the Aesthetic movement, an eclectic movement embracing many cultures and styles but emphasising, above all, the importance of art and good design in the home, became the dominant influence on interior design. Its principles were expounded in books such as Charles Locke Eastlake's influential *Hints on Household Taste* of 1868 and *The House Beautiful* by Clarence Cook, published in New York in 1881. In New York, the catalogue of the J.L. Mott Iron Works of 1888 featured an expensively fitted bathroom in the 'Elizabethan' style. A sixteenth-century feel to the room was created by enclosing the fittings in ornate wood panelling, which provided decorative unity to the fittings while hiding unsightly pipes from view. They also illustrated several bathroom interiors with plenty of carved wood panelling, stained glass and decorative tiles in what they called the 'Eastlake design'.[21] Choices of wood included mahogany, pine,

A 'modern bathroom in the Pompeian style' by Hampton and Sons, Pall Mall, London, 1894. (*Russell-Cotes Art Gallery and Museum*)

walnut or oak, although mahogany was the most popular and most suitable, being a close-grained wood that could withstand the humid climate of a bathroom. From the mid-1870s imposing combined plunge and shower baths, enclosed in wood panelling, became fashionable in the most expensive bathrooms. The shower canopy – an upright enclosure at the foot of the bath – usually consisted of a round arched opening flanked by fluted pilasters and topped with a heavy cornice. They looked more like a sixteenth-century pulpit or throne than a bath. The effect was to evoke a world of Renaissance popes and princes. The trade names, in some cases, further underlined the association: thus Twyfords introduced the 'Florentine' style decoration for some of their water closets in 1886 and the 'Cardinal' washstand in 1887. This mahogany cabinet was fitted with a tiled splash panel and the tiles, decorated in a deep orange and blue on white, recalled Italian 'majolica' (tin-glazed) earthenware of the sixteenth century. Thomas Twyford had one fitted in his own bathroom at Moor House, Bidulph in Staffordshire.

The impact of the Aesthetic movement on the bathroom was particularly apparent in the widespread adoption of tiles. They formed an ideal surface in the bathroom: they were at once decorative and highly functional providing a hard-wearing, water-resistant surface. Tin-glazed earthenware – or delftware – tiles had been popular in the eighteenth century, especially for the interiors of fireplaces, but had gone out of fashion by 1800. Tile manufacture was then revived after 1840 following a series of innovations which made possible the production of cheap, decorative tiles. In 1840 Richard Prosser patented a new technique for making articles from pressed clay, and this was soon adapted to the manufacture of tiles by Herbert Minton (1793–1858). The decorative possibilities of tiles

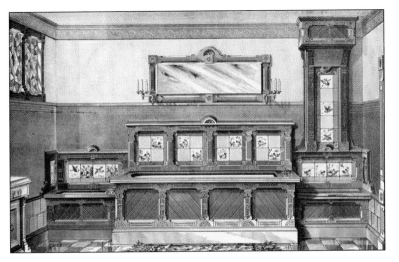

An 'Eastlake Design' bathroom by the J.L. Mott Iron Works Co., New York, 1888. The decorative scheme contains all the components that conformed with Eastlake's views on interior design, including the heavily ornate timberwork, the stained glass in the window and the hand-painted tiles in the panels behind the fittings. The heavily disguised water closet is on the left, the 'porcelain' or cast-iron bath in the centre and a foot or child's bath on the right.

was then increased in 1850 when Mintons introduced the use of opaque enamels that they called 'majolica'. Also in 1850 they devised a method of transfer printing.[22] Their majolica tiles were used the following year in the Alhambra Court at the Great Exhibition, and the same year transfer-printed tiles were used for the walls of the smoking room in the House of Commons. The wide range of decorative effects and designs the manufacturers were now able to produce – tiles with flowers, pastoral scenes, Japanese and Persian-inspired patterns and many others – fitted perfectly with the theories of good taste formulated by the Aesthetic Movement in the 1860s and 1870s. In 1867 Eastlake recommended the use of tiles in hallways[23] and from the early 1870s the use of tiles in the home rapidly increased just as the bathroom itself was becoming more common. New firms appeared such as Godwins and Maw and Co. of Shropshire, who were to become the largest manufacturers of tiles in the world by the 1890s. In reaction to the mass-produced product of the Staffordshire makers, William de Morgan (1838–1917) began making hand-made tiles from plastic clay in 1872. After 1875 he introduced the famous Persian tiles, which were hand painted in deep purples, blues and greens in imitation of the 'Isnik' designs of the sixteenth and seventeenth centuries, and these were used in some bathrooms.[24] Tiles were exported worldwide. Large quantities were shipped to America. At the Centennial Exposition staged at Philadelphia in 1876 the displays of the English manufacturers stimulated the growth of an American tile industry which evolved its own distinctive techniques and quickly established a reputation for a quality product.

The application of tiles in bathrooms ranged from matching panels behind the bath and washbasin to floors and the lining of entire walls. Schemes for tiled walls in the 1870s and 1880s usually followed the practice revived by the Aesthetic Movement of dividing the wall horizontally into dado, filling and frieze. The height of the dado varied – sometimes it was placed high – and the tiles used for the skirting, dado and frieze were frequently moulded in high relief in imitation of their wooden equivalents; these tiles were also often glazed in strong colours and patterns, deep yellows, for example, browns and even black – which contrasted with the lighter shades and simpler patterns of the filling. The overall effect could be sombre, which accorded with the subdued colour schemes favoured by followers of the Aesthetic Movement. Few tiled bathrooms were as magnificent – or quite as original – as that installed in 1885 at Gledhow Hall, Leeds by the owner, James Kitson (1835–1911), a manufacturer of steam locomotives. It was designed by Leeds architects, Chorley and Connon, who created a richly decorated

'The special feature in this room is that as far as possible the entire surface of the walls and ceilings is covered with glazed porcelain so as to ensure the utmost degree of cleanliness.'
The Builder reviewing the bathroom at Gledhow Hall, Leeds, 1885.

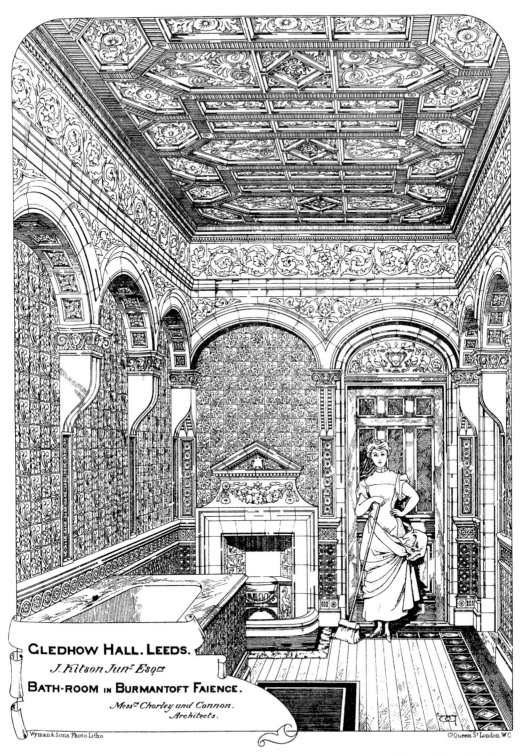

GLEDHOW HALL. LEEDS.
J. Kitson Junr Esqr
BATH-ROOM IN BURMANTOFT FAIENCE.
Messrs Chorley and Connon.
Architects.
Wyman & Sons. Photo-Litho.
Cr Queen St London. WC

The bathroom at Gledhow Hall, the home of the Leeds industrialist, James Kitson, which was designed by the Leeds architects, Chorley and Connon, and lined with 'Burmantoft Faience' made by Wilcox and Co. *The Builder*, 18 July 1885.

interior that included a series of moulded arches resting on vaguely
Ionic capitals above the bath. The joinery of the windows and doors
was in mahogany and walnut, but virtually every other surface was
finished in the heavily embossed, glossy 'Burmantofts faience' made
in Leeds by Wilcox and Co. The colour scheme was elaborate though
somewhat muted: browns and creams, greens and light yellows predominated.[25] Kitson enjoyed entertaining – Gladstone was a
frequent visitor – and this bathroom was clearly designed to impress.

Of course, it was wealthy industrialists and financiers – like
Kitson – and aristocrats who had the money to employ architects to
create opulent bathrooms. At Cardiff Castle, the architect, William
Burgess, created an exotic bathroom in the Moorish style for the
bachelor apartments of the Marquess of Bute in 1868.[26] In Bristol Sir
George White (1854–1916), who had made a fortune running the
city's trams and buses and established the British and Colonial
Aeroplane Company in 1910, lavished a fortune on Cotham House
between 1889 and 1915. He employed the leading Bristol architect,
Sir George Oatley, to refit and furnish his home. Notwithstanding
his progressive ideas (as early as 1912 he had realised that fighter
aircraft were to play a vital role in future warfare) his preference in
furniture was for new pieces but in a period style.[27] The two
bathrooms at Cotham House – the principal bedroom had its own *en
suite* – were furnished in the neo-classical manner. The walls were
heavily panelled in mahogany, which extended to the shower bath,
while the washbasin was recessed in a shell hood canopy. No pipes
were visible – even the toilet flush was activated by pressing a button
in the panelling. There were fireplaces and the floors were thickly
carpeted: comfort and luxury were very much in evidence.
Eighteenth-century classicism found its way into other bathrooms in
the 1890s and early 1900s. In Doulton's 1904 catalogue, the most
expensive bathroom scheme was fitted out in the Adam style.[28]

While such bathrooms, architect-designed and expensively
furnished, demand our attention, they were hardly typical. The
bathrooms built in cheaper housing between the 1870s and the early
1900s were simply furnished. Few survive in anything like their
original form, although the bathroom at 7 Blyth Grove in Worksop,
a semi-detached tradesman's house, built between 1905 and 1907
and now preserved by the National Trust, is probably typical.[29]
Lower down the social scale the bathroom was generally a small
room: there was less money to spend on fittings and furnishings and
so 'taste' was less evident. At 7 Blyth Grove, there were no extra
comforts, the bare walls were painted with oil paint for ease of
cleaning and as in many small bathrooms there was no fireplace.
Instead, paraffin stoves, which became popular in the 1870s, could

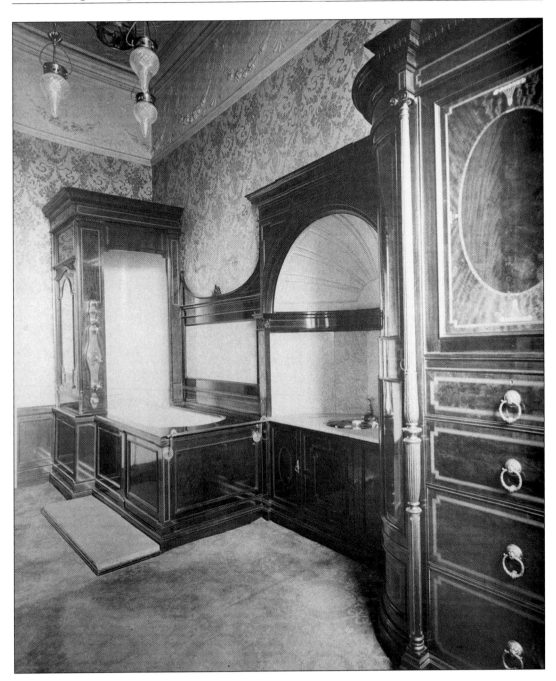

be used to heat the chimneyless room. An 1884 advertisement for the Albion Lamp Co. shows the corner of an unpretentious bathroom, simply furnished with a cast-iron bath sporting, however, one of their oil stoves.[30] For the occupant of a modest 1890s villa – perhaps in a terrace – but with a small upstairs bathroom, simply having hot and cold water was a luxury. Superfluous luxuries in the room were unnecessary and, moreover, undesirable. The scientific

The bathroom at Cotham House, Cotham, Bristol, the home of Sir George White, showing the cabinet washbasin in its alcove and canopy bath installed some time after 1889, shown in about 1915.
(*Sir George White*)

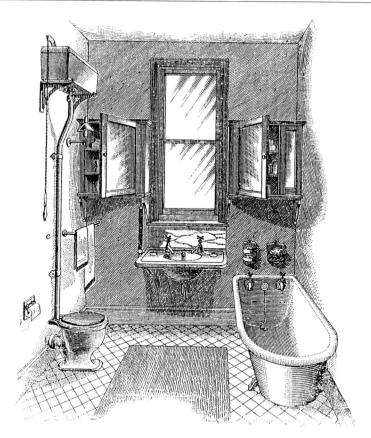

The plain and simple interior of a bathroom suitable for a house costing about £750 – a lower-middle-class house – in 1905. The bath is of cast iron and porcelain-enamelled on the inside rim and metallic-enamelled outside; it has brass screw-down globe taps. The white glazed earthenware lavatory is supported on white enamelled iron brackets and fitted with screw-down taps. The pedestal wash-down water closet is made of glazed fireclay and has a wooden ring seat and cover; the cistern is porcelain-enamelled cast iron.

discoveries of the previous half-century had established beyond all doubt the connection between dirt and disease, and high standards of cleanliness in the bathroom were expected. Their parlours may have been stuffed with furniture, fabrics and fussy ornament, but the bathroom was a room of hard bright surfaces. Anything which might harbour dirt such as wood panelling, rugs and carpets – and ornament – were condemned as insanitary. By the early 1900s, the day of the wood-panelled bathroom was over. It was this simpler style that Muthesius observed approvingly in 1904. 'If ornamental accessories are kept out of the bathroom,' he wrote, 'a truly modern character will be achieved.'[31] He likened a modern bathroom to a piece of 'scientific sculpture' where the aesthetic satisfaction came from an appreciation of 'form which has evolved exclusively out of purpose'. In the Edwardian bathroom, floral ornament and strong colours withered and died and relief and moulded ornament soon went the same way. By 1914 many bathrooms were clean and functional, but perhaps a little chilly. No wonder some mourned the passing of the cosy bath taken in front of the bedroom fire.

'If ornamental accessories are kept out of the bathroom, a truly modern character will be achieved.'
Herman Muthesius, 1904–5.

CHAPTER SIX

Essential Fittings and Expensive Fads

fitted baths and washbasins

In September 1886, reviewing sanitary appliances on view at the Edinburgh International Exhibition the trade journal, *The Ironmonger*, reported 'the rapid strides that have been made during the last few years in improving and perfecting this important branch of dwelling house fixtures'.[1] In the last quarter of the nineteenth century, as the bathroom itself consolidated its place in the home, and ideas on its furnishing developed, its three principal components – the bath, washbasin and water closet – were constantly being refined and improved. Between 1860 and 1899 over 3,500 patents were taken out to make sanitaryware easier to use and more comfortable, more economical in their use of water – and also safer: a constant worry of the water companies was contamination of mains water by foul water from poorly designed and fitted appliances. The principal aim, of course, was to make the fittings more sanitary – that is, cleaner – and in the last fifteen years or so of the nineteenth century, the introduction of simpler, free-standing fittings complemented the trend towards plainer bathroom interiors.

Expensively furnished bathrooms in the late nineteenth century were often fitted with plumbed-in sitz baths, bidets and separate shower and spray baths, but the basic fitting at all social levels was the bath. After the myriad variety of mid-Victorian portable baths, the fixed version settled down to being a full-length tub usually between 5 and 6 ft long inside; with running hot water, there was, after all, no longer any practical obstacle to filling a full-length bath. There were many detailed variations in the placing of the taps, waste and overflow, but the only major difference was between the parallel-sided – or 'equal-ended' – bath, as it was termed in the trade, and the tapered model which held less water. There was a greater range of materials. Many were made like portable baths of tinned or galvanised sheet iron and were lined in the same way with a japanned or enamelled surface often in imitation of a light-coloured marble. The exterior was not normally visible. Fixed sheet-metal baths were usually supported in a cradle that was boxed in with wooden panelling. The ends of the bath were curved to provide a comfortable back rest, but reclining in these baths was not easy as there was invariably an awkward angle between the sides, the back and base that was usually flat. In 1884 the London bath makers, R. Perkins, introduced a new style of bath at the International Health Exhibition at South Kensington. This bath, made of sheet copper and steel, had a gradual slope and a rounding of the bottom.[2] Several other established makers brought improved sheet-metal baths of copper and wrought steel in this decade, and all were clearly a response to a rival that was rapidly gaining ground – the cast-iron bath.[3]

Cast-iron baths were not a 'novelty' of the 1880s. They had been produced by iron founders as early as the 1850s. William Bennett, iron founders, kitchen-range and grate manufacturers in Liverpool, were advertising their cast-iron baths in 1859,[4] and in the early 1900s, Miltons of Falkirk and Glasgow claimed over fifty years' experience as manufacturers of cast-iron baths.[5] Cast iron had been used extensively for the production of domestic goods – grates, ovens and cooking utensils – or 'hollow-ware' since the late eighteenth century. A hard, durable and impervious metal, it was easily cast into intricate shapes in large sizes, and therefore ideal for the making of baths. Cast-iron baths could be made in one piece with a smooth contoured interior surface. Moreover, they were cheap.

Doubtless encouraged by the increasing popularity of baths, other iron founders entered the field. By the 1870s T. and C. Clark and Co. of Wolverhampton were making cast-iron baths lined with 'porcelain' enamel.[6] Clarks could trace their business back to 1795 when they had begun the manufacture of hollow-ware – pots, kettles and pans – and in 1839 they had pioneered in Britain the German process of applying porcelain enamel to cast-iron cooking utensils.[7] The enamel consisted of a hard, siliceous glaze which was applied at a high temperature so that it became practically fused into the metal. The resulting smooth and lustrous white surface provided the perfect interior for baths. A cheaper interior finish was metallic enamelling. This was simply enamel paint and was the finish commonly

By the late nineteenth century, in response to the growth at the lower end of the market, manufacturers introduced cheaper products like this free-standing cast-iron bath introduced by Morrison, Ingram and Co., Manchester, in 1890. The bath had a hot and cold supply, an earthenware soap dish and lift-up waste at the foot end. According to *The Ironmonger*, this inexpensive bath was 'especially fitted for ordinary dwelling house property'. *The Ironmonger*, 27 December 1890. (*Rural History Centre*)

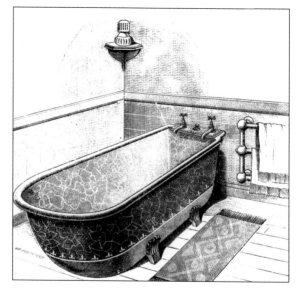

applied to sheet-metal baths: it could be applied to represent marble or other types of decoration, but it was not as durable. Every few years the bath interior would require repainting, although few would have wished to follow Pooter, the London clerk, in choosing red.

By 1904, Doulton and Co. claimed that vitreous enamel had almost entirely superseded the paint or metallic finish.[8] Facing stiff competition from the iron founders, the sheet-metal bath makers fought back: they emphasised the disadvantages of cast iron, that it was heavy and brittle and that it chilled the water. The weight and fragility of cast-iron baths in transit was a problem within the trade, but for the consumer the vitreous enamel cast-iron bath was comfortable to recline in, easy to keep clean and affordable. And as for the tendency of cast iron to absorb the heat, the solution was to line the bath with porcelain enamel. So when, for example, the Cannon Hollow-ware Co. of Deepfields, near Bilston, Staffordshire introduced their non-conductive 'porceliron' bath lining in 1897 they made much of the fact that 'one filling effectually warms the bath'.[9]

> *'Painted the bath red, and was delighted with the result. Sorry to say Carrie was not, in fact we had a few words about it . . . She said she had never heard of such a thing as a bath being painted red. I replied: It's merely a matter of taste.'*
> Mr Pooter, 1892.

John Shanks (1825–95)

JOHN SHANKS began life as a plumber in relatively humble circumstances, but was to establish one of the leading sanitaryware companies in Britain. He was the son of a handloom weaver in Paisley and was apprenticed as a plumber to Wallace and Connell of Glasgow. He worked as a journeyman plumber in the Paisley area until the mid-1850s when he established his own plumbing business in Barrhead, 7 miles south-west of Glasgow. The firm began on a small site in Main Street, employing eight people.

His first patent in 1863 featured a trapless water closet, which became the company's 'Number Four' and brought them sales nationwide. In 1875 he founded Shanks and Co., Sanitary Engineers, with his brother Andrew, who was also a plumber, and the firm expanded rapidly. They added an iron foundry to their works about this time, and in 1878 introduced the 'Independent' cast-iron bath with integral shelf, waste and overflow. By the 1890s the firm occupied a 7-acre site and employed 600 men. All stages of the production of sanitaryware were completed on the Main Street site, from iron moulding to enamelling: some twenty different trades were involved.

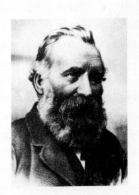

John Shanks. (*Mitchell Library, Glasgow*)

John Shanks showed considerable business acumen and technical skill. He recognised the potential of sanitaryware at a time when public awareness of the importance of public health and increased personal hygiene was growing. He was a prolific inventor, taking out some 100 patents by 1894. He took pride in the company's reputation for producing reliable, durable and reasonably priced goods which were found in hospitals and public buildings throughout Britain. They also supplied fittings to passenger liners including the *Lusitania* and the *Titanic*, and exported to many countries overseas, ensuring the company a worldwide reputation. Shanks married twice, and his son John with his nephew William carried on the business after his death in December 1895. The firm continued to flourish, adding the Victorian Pottery at Barrhead in about 1902. Shanks remained a household name in connection with bathroom fittings into the twenty-first century.

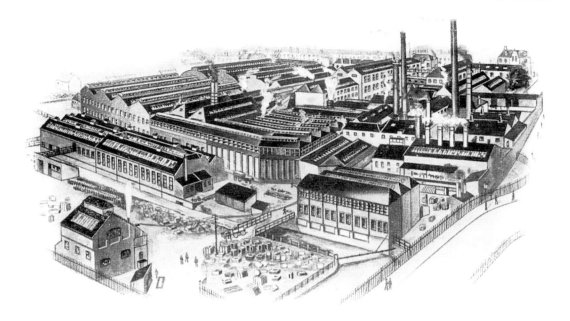

Cast-iron baths, of course, were a basic product of some of the leading sanitaryware manufacturers. Shanks of Barrhead, near Glasgow, added an iron foundry to their works in the mid-1870s, and in 1878 introduced their 'Independent' bath with integral shelf, waste and overflow. The company was founded by John Shanks (1826–95) who had started business as a plumber in Paisley in 1851, moving to Barrhead two years later. By the 1890s the firm was established as one of the leading sanitaryware manufacturers in Britain, employing 600 men at their seven-acre factory site, the Tubal Works.[10] In 1883, Shanks's agent in Manchester, Alexander Finlay Morrison, set up his own company in partnership with Mathew Ingram. Within four years they were employing 120 men at the Hygiea Works, a short distance from Manchester Docks in the Cornbrooke district of the city where all their fittings, except the earthenware goods, were made.[11] The potters, Doulton and Co., already renowned for their stoneware sanitary goods, extended their operations to include the manufacture of cast-iron baths and other metal sanitaryware in 1888 when they established an iron foundry at Paisley.[12] These and other leading companies made much of the upper end of their range – the opulent and expensive shower baths and washstands – exhibiting them at trade fairs at home and abroad and featuring them in full colour in their sumptuous trade catalogues. Occasionally they attracted aristocratic and even royal patronage. Royal warrants brought prestige and for Henry Doulton, a knighthood, but it was the 'bread and butter' articles – particularly

The extensive Tubal Works of Shanks and Co., Barrhead, near Glasgow, in 1907, which were named after the Old Testament figure, Tubal Cain, the first worker in brass and iron. This was a period of expansion for the company. The Victorian Pottery had opened a few years previously and in 1918 Shanks acquired J. and M. Craig, sanitaryware potters in Kilmarnock, established in 1831. (*Mitchell Library, Glasgow*)

the cheap cast-iron bath – that formed the basis of their commercial success, while bringing, at the same time, a new level of hygiene and sanitary comfort to the masses.

The cheapest baths required a wooden enclosure like the sheet-metal baths but the cast-iron bath came into its own in the 1880s and 1890s as a free-standing tub. From the early 1880s, the wood panelling enclosing baths and washbasins was condemned by sanitarians and some architects. It was, they claimed, unhygienic and harboured dirt and disease. The change in fashion was apparent on both sides of the Atlantic. In 1886, an American architect, Glenn Brown, reported in *The Builder* that 'it is fast becoming a common practice in this country to dispense with all wooden panelling, boxing and casing around water closets, bath tubs and wash-basins'.[13] Enclosed wooden fittings remained popular through the 1880s, but by the early 1890s a change in fashion was apparent as manufacturers turned to making open, free-standing fittings. By 1904 Muthesius could write, 'in good bathrooms of the past the bath used to be encased in wood but the custom has now ceased entirely'.[14] It was now possible to clean under the bath. Muthesius also noted that the attached wooden rim around the top of the bath was fast disappearing. These had been necessary to protect the enamel along the thin top edge of the bath, but by the late 1880s manufacturers such as Shanks had introduced the rolled edge top, which continued the enamelled interior outwards over a continuous, wide-curving rim.[15] The wooden surround was no longer necessary and another obstacle to absolute cleanliness around the bath was removed.

The exterior of the bath now became a focus for decoration. The feet were variously cast as clawed feet, acanthus leaves or with other designs derived from Greek and Roman furniture styles. The link with antiquity was also conveyed through some of the designs in metallic enamels on the bath sides and also through some of the trade names. Inspired by Archimedes's success in solving problems while soaking in the bath, Shanks had their patent 'Eureka' plunge bath while Morrison, Ingram and Co. named two of their models the 'Cleopatra' and the 'Empress'. Tapered baths were sometimes described as 'Roman' baths. Other enamelled designs featured garlands of roses, vine leaves and formal swags. Shanks's 'Fin de Siecle' bath of 1899 was available in sixteen different patterns, including a whimsical arrangement of scroll-like waves and flying dolphins repeated in a band below the waist. Strong colour combinations were popular: emerald greens and bright blues were matched with 'old gold'; black was combined with deep reds – and more 'old gold' – or silvery greys; but for those with conservative

'It is usual to case the bath with framed and panelled woodwork, but this would be better omitted in order that the space under and around the bath may be visible and kept clean.' Percival Smith and Keith Young, architects, 1883.

tastes, the manufacturers supplied plenty of sombre wood-grained and marbled finishes.

In the 1890s the price of the cheapest cast-iron baths compared favourably with a sheet-metal gas bath. A simple unadorned tub, 5 ft 6 in long without accessories could be purchased for as little as £1 13s, while a 'General Gordon' gas bath could be had for £6 7s 6d. Rolled-edge porcelain-enamelled baths were more than twice as much, costing around £15, which placed them in the middle price range.[16] More expensive again were the so-called porcelain baths which were actually made from carefully prepared fireclay that because it was porous was given a pottery glaze, which the manufacturers called 'porcelain enamel'. Fireclay was the cheapest type of ceramicware, but by associating it with porcelain the manufacturers aimed to give it an air of luxury. The finished surface resembled fine china and was given various trade names such as 'Queen's Ware' and 'Victorian Ware'. The making of fireclay baths originated in Stourbridge in the 1850s. Francis T. Rufford of Stourbridge won the Gold Isis Medal of the Society of Arts, sponsored by Prince Albert, for making the first one-piece fireclay bath in 1850.[17] Soon fireclay baths were being made in Scotland and Yorkshire. James Kitson's sumptuous, tiled bathroom at Gledhow Hall, Leeds, completed in 1885, was fitted with a porcelain bath. The 1888 catalogue of the American company, J.L. Mott Ironworks, featured a porcelain bath, moulded in one piece, which was proudly claimed to be 'without doubt the finest piece of ware that has yet been produced of so large a size by any potter'.[18] Thomas W. Twyford (1849–1921) in Hanley, Stoke on Trent, and one of the leading sanitaryware potters, began manufacturing fireclay sanitaryware in

'Rufford's or Finch's porcelain baths are clean and durable'.
S. Stevens Hellyer, 1877.

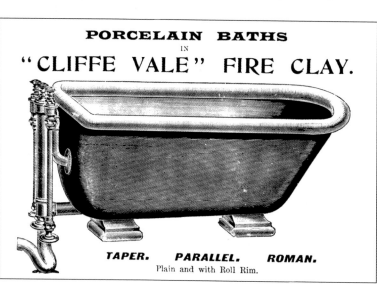

PORCELAIN BATHS
IN
"CLIFFE VALE" FIRE CLAY.

TAPER.   PARALLEL.   ROMAN.
Plain and with Roll Rim.

Twyford's Cliffe Vale 'porcelain'-enamelled fireclay bath from an advertisement of 1898. Twyfords began to manufacture fireclay as opposed to earthenware in the early 1890s. Unlike earthenware, fireclay products were fired just once and the glaze applied directly on to the clay. However, the drying and applying of several coats of glaze took between ten and twelve weeks for a large bath like this. Fireclay baths had a very solid, comfortable appearance due to the thick body of clay used.
The Ironmonger, 21 May 1898.
(*Rural History Centre*)

the early 1890s.[19] He had a fireclay bath made for his home, Whitmore Hall, Whitmore, near Newcastle-under-Lyme, Staffordshire in 1896, which, remarkably, has survived and is now on display at Twyford's own museum of sanitaryware at Alsager, Cheshire. Shanks and Co. started making their own fireclay goods from 1902 following the building of the Victorian Pottery at Barrhead. Porcelain-enamelled fireclay baths were expensive: Doulton's model of 1904 cost £25 12s.[20] The same year Muthesius said, 'porcelain baths are the most popular and have entirely replaced others', but he must have immediately realised this was not entirely true and added, 'the enamelled cast-iron bath is frequently used in cheaper bathrooms'.[21]

'Bath tubs in the USA vary little from bath tubs in England.' Glenn Brown, American architect, 1886.

Thomas William Twyford (1849–1921)

T HE TWYFORDS had been involved in potting in north Staffordshire since the seventeenth century. In 1849 Thomas Twyford had turned almost exclusively to the manufacture of sanitaryware at new works at Bath Street, Hanley. Upon his untimely death at the age of forty-six, his son, Thomas William Twyford, found himself in charge of the family business.

The business expanded rapidly with a second pottery, the Abbey Works, at Bucknall, Stoke-on-Trent in production by 1875, and then in 1887 the Cliffe Vale works was established. This occupied 9 acres of land alongside the Bridgewater Canal, Hanley. Twyford paid particular attention to the welfare of his employees in the design of these works, building spacious, well ventilated workshops to reduce the risk of pneumoconiosis – 'potters' asthma' – caused by the inhalation of fine sharp particles of silica dust. Twyford then brought some experienced fireclay potters from Scotland to Hanley, and by late 1890 had added 'porcelain enamelled' fireclay articles to his range of goods. Further expansion in the early twentieth century saw the opening of a factory at Ratingen, near Dusseldorf, Germany to avoid high German import duties. In 1911 new fireclay works were built opposite the Cliffe Vale site, and the following year a new pottery was established at Etruria.

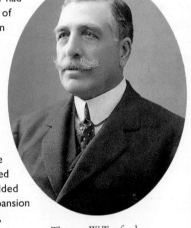

Thomas W. Twyford.
(*Twyford Bathrooms*)

By the late nineteenth century Twyford's were indisputably the largest makers of ceramic sanitaryware in the Staffordshire pottery towns and one of the leading makers in the country with a worldwide reputation. Twyford always ensured that his products represented the latest thinking in sanitaryware, yet his role as an innovator may have previously been over-emphasised. Although he took out thirteen patents for sanitaryware between 1884 and 1892, none of the major, lasting developments of this period can be attributed to him. Thus the 'Unitas', while being one of the earliest fully enclosed pedestal wash-out closets, was not the first: it was preceded by George Jennings's 'Pedestal Vase'. But if Twyford lacked Jennings's originality, neither did he make his mistakes and the majority of Twyfords' products were extremely successful. They were, besides, some of the most aesthetically pleasing, and the range of decorative ceramic sanitaryware illustrated in colour in his highly ornate *Twentieth Century Catalogue* of 1901 arguably represents one of the all-time peaks in sanitaryware design. Today, as Twyford Bathrooms, based at Alsager, Cheshire, the company maintains its position as a major producer of ceramic sanitaryware.

The most expensive and luxurious fitted baths in the late nineteenth century were the canopy baths, which in the 1890s ranged in price from about £35 to £50. Consisting of an enclosure containing various shower and spray effects fixed to a full-length bath, they emerged in the 1870s as the successors to the portable-shower baths of the early and mid-nineteenth century, but as they were connected to a pressurised water supply, their performance was vastly superior. No longer limited by the quantity of water held in the overhead cistern, bathers could enjoy a powerful shower and needle spray for as long as they wished. In expensive bathrooms they made imposing centre-pieces, the sentry box-like enclosure at the foot of the bath standing over 7 ft high. Smeaton and Sons of London were the first makers to patent an enclosed canopy bath in 1874.[22] It was subsequently named the 'Imperial' needle bath and put on show at the Paris Exhibition in 1878.[23] Within this impressive mahogany-clad fitting, bathers could have a conventional soak relaxing in the full-length bath, or alternatively stand within the enclosure and subject themselves to the more invigorating experiences of shower, douche and needle spray. They were soon being made by other leading makers including Shanks, Doulton, Morrison, Ingram and Co. The best models included a shower spray and a powerful torrent of water – the douche – from above, a needle spray from tiny perforations in the sides, an ascending spray and a thin sheet of water delivered from a wide but shallow slit in the side of the bath. But not everyone was impressed: in 1891, S. Stevens Hellyer, a leading London manufacturer and sanitary reformer dismissed the combination of effects as, 'nothing more than fads'.[24]

Using one of these baths for the first time may well have been a daunting experience. To control the various water effects and their temperature, the bather had to work a set of valves usually located on the side edge of the canopy. They had as many as five valves: two lettered hot and cold which controlled the water supply and then valves for the needle bath, shower or supply to the bath. The needle and shower could be used together or separately. Morrison, Ingram and Co.'s 'Oriental' plunge and shower bath of 1886 introduced a dividing and regulating lever to select various temperatures of water for the bath and the other outlets. This arrangement reduced the plumbing work by two-thirds and as *The Ironmonger* reported in 1886, 'the whole arrangement of the hot, tepid and cold water supply is greatly simplified'.[25]

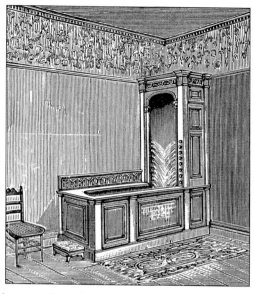

The 'Imperial' needle bath patented by Smeaton and Sons, London, in 1874, was the first enclosed canopy bath combining shower and plunge bath. The bath is enclosed in wood panelling and the various water effects, including needle, shower or douche, could be selected by adjusting the pull-out knobs at the side.

'The Independent Oriental Bath . . . is designed to afford a refreshing and invigorating bath, giving perfect freedom to the user and obviating that sense of confinement experienced in the covered and darkened canopy baths.'
Morrison, Ingram and Co., 1887.

The vertical enclosure contained the complicated system of pipes that took water from the mains to the various outlets; it also rendered a shower curtain unnecessary. But the interior of earlier models like Smeaton's 'Imperial' was cramped, as the canopy was no wider than the bath. Shanks introduced a new shape to the bath tub to overcome this problem, widening the shower end to roughly three-quarters of a circle. The rest of the bath flared out from the narrowest point of the shower section ending in a wide curving back producing a keyhole-like shape. The more spacious canopy not only provided more elbow room but also ensured that the spray jets all converged to the centre. Shanks adopted this for their 'Eureka' and 'Independent' canopy baths and it was subsequently adopted by Doulton and other makers. Shanks exhibited the 'Eureka' canopy bath at the International Health Exhibition in South Kensington in 1884: fitted with the full range of shower effects and enclosed in an elegant wooden cabinet they described the 'Eureka' as 'the acme of luxurious bathing'.[26] But not everyone appreciated showering in an enclosed space, even if it was wider. So Shanks's 'Independent' plunge and spray bath, which was on show at the Edinburgh International Exhibition two years later, had a metal enclosure which was open at the top. The 'Independent' was also made with no enclosure, exposing the yards of nickel-plated pipe supplying the needle spray, douche and shower.[27] In 1886, Morrison, Ingram and Co. introduced a similar model, the 'Oriental Bath', which was open at the top; in this, they claimed, 'perfect freedom and comfort are afforded to the user without the sense of confinement which is inseparable from the ordinary covered over and darkened canopy'.[28] The replacement of the wood casing with canopies of sheet zinc or copper also reflected the growing unpopularity of wood in the bathroom. Finished in colourful stencilled designs, these magnificent all-metal fittings represented the ultimate in late Victorian bath design – 'fitted up', as S. Stevens Hellyer wryly observed in 1891, 'to suit the sweet wills and long purses of the rich'.[29]

Two of Shanks's 'Eureka' plunge and shower baths, fully enclosed in mahogany panelling, were installed at Kinloch Castle on the Isle of Rhum in 1901, although by then the fashion for grandiose shower baths was waning. Writing in 1904, Muthesius

'Combination baths, combining what many consider to be nothing more than fads, such as spray, sitz, douche and shower baths can be fitted up to suit the sweet wills and long purses of the rich.'
S. Stevens Hellyer, 1891.

Morrison, Ingram and Co.'s 'Oriental' spray bath, *c*. 1893. The bath was cast iron and the open-topped spray enclosure of galvanised iron. The plan on the left shows the 'key-hole' shape that was adopted from the mid-1880s. (*Thomas Crapper and Co. Ltd*)

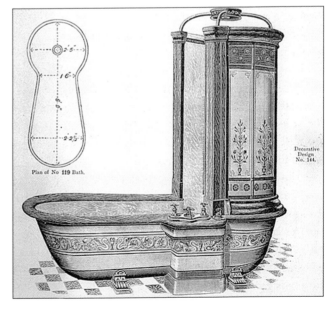

Plan of No 119 Bath.

Decorative Design No. 144.

said the present idea was to separate the bath from the shower. The separate shower was more compact than a canopy bath and, importantly, was considered more hygienic, as the same water never came into contact with the body more than once. Two London companies, Hayward Tyler and Co., of Whitecross Street and John Smeaton Son and Co. had their own versions on the market in 1890. Instead of being attached to a full-length bath tub, the open arrangement of pipes supplying needle, spray and douche was fixed to uprights screwed into a tiled floor. Whilst never common in private houses, many were fitted in public baths, private clubs and large hotels. Hayward Tyler supplied their needle douche bath to the Hamman Baths in Jermyn Street, close to Piccadilly. Smeaton claimed a long list of customers for their 'Carlsbad' bath which had six rows of needles, each controlled by a separate cock, including Camden Town Turkish Baths, the baths at Leamington Spa and the Hydro in Buxton. They had also supplied it to the Mont Doré Hotel in St Petersburg, the Hotel Imperial in Paris, and closer to home – the Royal Bath Hotel in Bournemouth.[30] In about 1900 they were recommended for expensive private bathrooms. Doulton's catalogue for 1904 shows a 'top of the range' bathroom furnished with a glazed fireclay bath and separate needle shower.[31] By the early 1900s, simpler showers consisting of an overhead shower rose over a square 'safe' or well with a drain were becoming the most popular choice.[32]

From 'Paris s'amuse' of 1897, an elegant Parisienne showers in a combined needle and overhead shower consisting of open pipework. (*Mary Evans Picture Library*)

Plumbed-in bidets, sitz and foot baths were also made for 'bathrooms intended to be very complete in their appointments'. Sitz baths were similar to portable hip baths, which meant the bather's feet rested on the floor: Shanks's model of the 1880s looked rather like an armchair of galvanised iron without legs. Bidets – for 'baths of a special nature' – had appeared in France by the early eighteenth century.[33] The characteristic violin-shaped bowl was kept in a dressing stand or night table along with the chamber pot. The late nineteenth-century version was a free-standing earthenware pedestal bowl with its own plumbing. By the mid-1880s, Shanks were advertising their 'Patent Pedestal Bidet' with hot and cold water and an ascending spray: they claimed 'it is a very necessary appliance in a well appointed bathroom'. Unfortunately, manufacturers like Shanks promoted the bidet but failed to explain it. This continental appliance was little understood and even mistrusted in Britain and America. Perhaps it looked just a little too much like the pedestal water closet which also appeared in the 1880s. On occasions bidets have been used in error as water closets by visitors ignorant of their true purpose: perhaps the ultimate social 'faux pas'.

Even when the function of the bidet was understood, a lack of space and the expense were enough to restrict its use. The same was true of foot and sitz baths and separate showers: after all, feet, hips and 'private parts' could be soaked just as effectively in a conventional bath. But no one doubted the importance of the lavatory washbasin, and as the fitted bathroom spread from the 1870s this became one of its standard fixtures. For washing hands and face, shampooing hair, cleaning teeth and for men, shaving beards and moustaches, the fitted washbasin was the natural successor to the free-standing washstand which had become a common article of furniture in many bedrooms and dressing rooms from the late eighteenth century. And the plumbed-in lavatories of the 1870s and 1880s were made to look like an item of furniture: they were usually enclosed in a marble-topped mahogany cabinet with an impressive, if fussy, back panel of decorative tiles, bevelled glass mirrors, jewel drawers and shelves surrounded with plenty of carved ornament.

The earliest washbasins were usually set into the top of the cabinet and were of two varieties: the tip-up basin, which had been introduced by George Jennings (1810–82), a London sanitary engineer, by 1851 and the plug basin. Basins were either made of enamelled iron[34] or earthenware. Tip-up basins were simple, cheap and effective and were widely used in the second half of the nineteenth century. They were mounted on pivots over an outer shell or receiver and the waste water was quickly dispatched by lifting the front rim which was often made with a projecting rim inscribed 'lift up'. One imposing cabinet lavatory introduced by the London firm, Smeaton and Sons, in 1878 combined a tip-up basin with a 'door action' urinal which was contained in a cupboard at the side of the

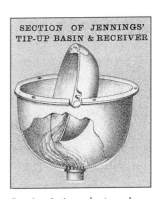

SECTION OF JENNINGS' TIP-UP BASIN & RECEIVER

Jennings's tip-up basin and receiver from Twyford's 1879 catalogue. (*Twyford Bathrooms*)

unit: when the door was opened tap water automatically flowed into the urinal until it was closed.[35] It was not long, however, before tip-up basins were being condemned by sanitary reformers such as S. Stevens Hellyer for being 'foul and filthy'. The problem was that the inner surfaces of the bowl and receiver accumulated soap and scum, which was then difficult to remove. George Jennings responded by introducing bowls which could be lifted out so that the inner surfaces could be thoroughly cleaned.[36] Other manufacturers, such as Doulton, followed his example, but by the early 1900s the day of the tip-up basin was nearly over.

Plug basins – as the name implied – contained an outlet with a plug in the bottom. Like tip-up basins they were often recessed into a marble top, but this was not an ideal arrangement as the joint between the earthenware basin and the marble top was rarely effective and inclined to leak. The marble itself was also prone to chipping and cracking. By the 1870s, the fixed lavatory basin had developed into an all-in-one earthenware fitting incorporating its own surround in the form of a slab, apron and skirting at the sides and back: Twyfords included a range of earthenware washbasins in their 1879 catalogue. The overall shape varied: some were square or rectangular but round-fronted and 'cornered' – with a three-sided front – were popular. Right-angled basins were also made to fit in corners, a useful consideration in smaller bathrooms. The slab usually contained recesses for soap at the sides, often prettily scalloped, while the bowl was usually round, oval or D-shaped. Some models, such as

'The basin I find easiest to use and most pleasant to use, tilts out the water by lifting a handle or rather a finger niche.' Florence Caddy, 1877.

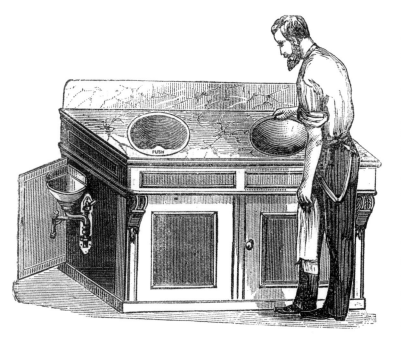

A combined tip-up washbasin and urinal introduced by Smeaton and Sons, London, in 1878. Water was obtained by gently pressing the front of the basin to obtain cold water and pressing a little harder to admit hot water. It was emptied by tipping the bowl upwards. Upon opening the side door water flowed into the urinal until the door closed. In 1878 *The Ironmonger* wrote, 'The luxurious manner in which they fit up some of their appliances has inaugurated quite a new era in domestic sanitary matters.' *The Ironmonger*, 19 October 1878. (*Rural History Centre*)

Shanks's 'Citizen' of the 1880s had a recess at the back of the bowl for the waste and overflow. Many basins were plain white, although they were also made with hand-painted or printed underglaze decoration in one or more colour or in gold. Blue and brown were popular single colours but some of the loveliest designs were the polychrome floral ones which often complemented the patterns of the tiles behind the basin, and from the early 1890s were made to match the water closet.

The elaborate cabinet lavatories, costing as much as £40 or £50, were the perfect companions to canopy baths in the more expensive bathrooms, but they were beyond the means of the lower-middle class who were rapidly adding bathrooms to their houses during the 1880s and 1890s. Simpler more affordable washbasins were needed to supply the widening market, and by about 1890 cast-iron lavatory stands had appeared costing typically between £5 and £10. George Jennings showed the way with his tip-up lavatory of 1881 which was supported on a simple metal stand, and in the mid-1880s Shanks's 'Patent Sanitary Lavatory' consisted of a fixed ceramic washbasin supported on wrought-iron scrolled brackets. The use of cast iron for furniture was not new: J.C. Loudon had been an enthusiastic exponent of iron furniture in the 1830s, and from the middle of the century, the manufacture of cast-iron bedsteads had expanded. Cast-iron garden furniture became popular, and in the 1860s and 1870s, treadle sewing machines, mangles, wringers and washing machines were made with decorative cast-iron supports. In the 1880s, small round tables resting on a cast-iron tripod base became fashionable in restaurants and public houses. The adoption of cast iron for lavatory stands, therefore, was almost inevitable.

In the early 1890s, Shanks advertised their 'New Patent Imperial Lavatory' which was fixed on an ornamental cast-iron stand with a japanned finish. Every part of the ironwork was cast with elaborate

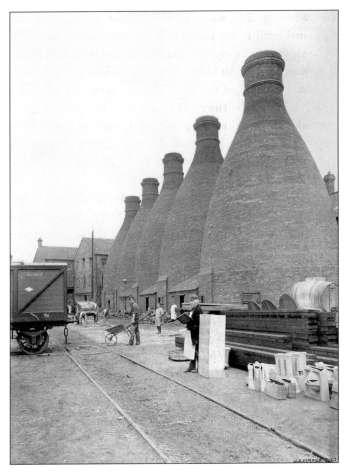

The glost ovens at Twyford's Cliffe Vale pottery, *c.* 1898. These were used for a second firing of earthenware to fix the glaze. (*Twyford Bathrooms*)

pierced and raised decoration: the side supports, the frame holding the basin and the back panel which incorporated a tiled back, shelf and bevelled plate-glass mirror. Shanks emphasised that 'this system of cast-iron lavatory stand combines artistic appearance with cheapness and sanitary value'. Twyfords said much the same thing about their 'Athena' lavatory – a similar unit introduced in 1892: it was 'artistic, strong, sanitary', they claimed. Many were made by iron founders in Glasgow, such as Watson Gow and Co., and Manchester firms such as Morrison, Ingram and Co. and Bennett's Ironfoundry Co. The cast-iron frames were embellished with a variety of designs, but swirling leaves and flowers were popular as were architectural motifs: Bennett's 'Louis' suite was made of Rococo-inspired asymmetrical curls, while Doulton's 'Improved Lavatories' of 1895 had a back panel framed by fluted pilasters and a broken pediment. Twyford's 'Athena' had winged angels – or perhaps they were gods – cast into the side brackets. The frame was coated in enamel paint – the best models being finished in several colours – thus the 'Louis XV' lavatory made by Morrison, Ingram and Co. was available in white, pale blue and gold. But the owner could paint the cast-iron work to match the colour scheme of their bathroom, or at least to match the colour of the other cast-iron articles of the 1890s bathroom: the sides of the bath and the brackets supporting the water-closet cistern and seat.

Cast-iron lavatory stands were ideal for smaller bathrooms. Not only were they cheaper than cabinet models, but they took up less space as the frame was usually little wider than the basin. Cast-iron stands were also considered more sanitary than enclosed washbasins. They did not harbour dirt and it was easier to clean underneath them. They were also easier for plumbers to 'get at' when repairs were necessary. With an eye on the export market the makers claimed one further advantage for cast iron: in tropical

A corner lavatory washbasin by Morrison, Ingram and Co., Manchester, 1887, with their 'noiseless and steamless' inlets, patented in 1883. Note the fan, a popular Arts and Crafts ornament, perched on the tile back. *The Ironmonger*, 1 October 1883. (*Rural History Centre*)

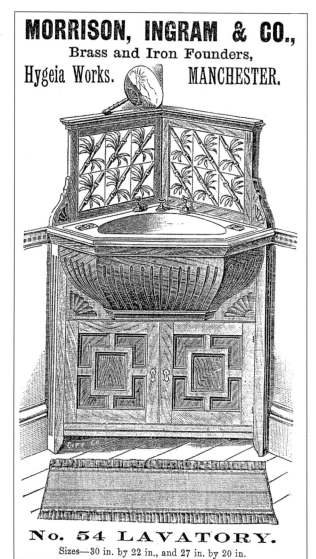

MORRISON, INGRAM & CO.,

Brass and Iron Founders,

Hygeia Works.   **MANCHESTER.**

No. 54 LAVATORY.

Sizes—30 in. by 22 in., and 27 in. by 20 in.

IN MAHOGANY, WALNUT OAK, or PITCH PINE.

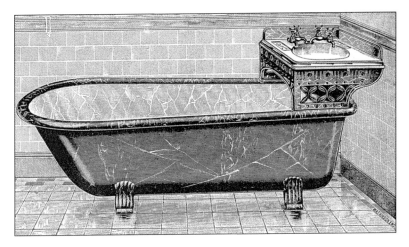

The 'Bramstone' cast-iron combination bath by Morrison, Ingram and Co., Manchester, 1895, with lavatory above supported by decorative cast-iron brackets. Such combinations saved on space and plumbing.

countries it was immune to damage from the damp of the rainy season and from termites, 'an energetic and abiding destroyer of everything made of wood'.[37] Catering for the growing demand for baths and washbasins in small houses with little space, in the 1880s manufacturers introduced combined baths and lavatories which consisted of a washbasin in a cast-iron frame attached to the top of the bath. The 'Cottage Bath' of T. and C. Clark made its debut at the Staffordshire Exhibition in July 1884: this combined bath and lavatory even had a hinged cover which could serve as an ironing board.[38] This bath, like any sanitary appliance attached to the name 'cottage', was aimed at the lower end of the market, and in the 1890s these combination baths with ornate cast-iron supports for the basin featured in many hardware catalogues. But fashions change, and in the early 1900s the elaborate cast-iron frame fell victim to a trend towards simpler furniture. Cast-iron ornament trapped dust and was time-consuming to clean. It was no longer regarded as 'artistic', and by 1910 all-ceramic pedestal washbasins had replaced cast-iron lavatories in the manufacturers' catalogues. Some were made of glazed fireclay – like the baths – and others of earthenware and some had Art Noveau-style decoration in relief on the exterior of the bowls and the pillar. They were white, plain and simple and eminently suited to the Edwardian sanitary bathroom.

Bathroom fittings connected to piped water required valves to control the supply. In 1865 Samuel Timmins, a Birmingham industrialist, wrote of the impact of recent sanitary improvements and 'the modern luxury of the bath' on the design of taps.[39] The brass founders and specialist cock founders, involved in the making of cocks and taps of all kinds, introduced the screw-down compression tap which was capable of withstanding the pressure of the

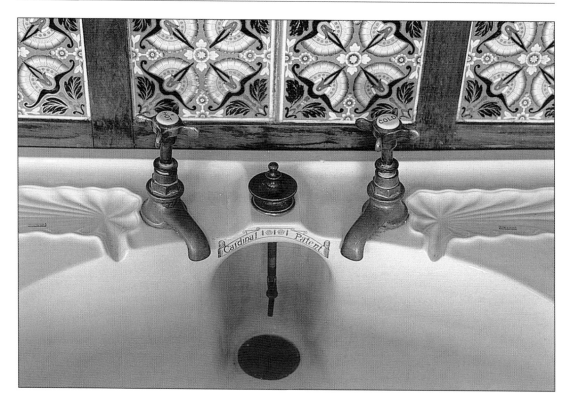

water in the mains.[40] Traditionally, water cocks were made of pot metal – a high lead/copper alloy which was a drab grey colour, but the founders introduced 'yellow metal' for the making of kitchen and bathroom taps. This was a type of brass containing as much lead as zinc and a small amount of tin. In this more attractive metal, which could take a polish, pillar taps attached to the bath or basin by a lock nut became a handsome component of the fitting. Baths were often made with 'globe' taps that were fitted to the vertical side of the bath. The cheapest taps were left untreated and these required constant polishing to stay bright; better-quality ones were lacquered and by the 1870s nickel-plated taps were also available. For the very 'best work', taps were also offered with silver or even platinum plating. The cross handle used to turn the tap was sometimes engraved with the words 'hot' and 'cold', and by 1880 white ceramic inserts in the tops with the same words printed in black or gold had become popular.

By the 1880s many patents had been taken out for more elaborate valves for baths and basins. Quick-action taps were made by 1880: these had a larger internal screw and were operated by a lever one turn of which was enough to open or close the supply. Cam-action taps, which were operated by a thumb lever, were also being made by the 1880s, and in 1881 the Birmingham makers, Martineau and

Twyford's 'Cardinal' washbasin with its original brass pillar taps with ceramic inlays.

Smith, advertised self-closing bath valves made with lift-up pulls attached by chains to a counterweight which controlled the valve.[41] In 1889, Llewellins and James, the leading brass founders in Bristol, advertised a set of interlocking bath valves that had a catch attached to the waste so that it could not be opened until the supply was shut off, thus preventing water being wasted.[42]

Various patents were taken out to get around the inconvenience of the nozzles of the taps projecting over the edge of the bath or basin. In 1877, John Shanks took out a patent for delivering water to basins through side inlets or a passage with a bottom slit located near the bottom.[43] Shanks used a similar design in the 1880s on their 'Citizen' washbasins and 'Imperial' baths. Only the spindle and knobs of the tap were exposed and the water entered the basin through small perforations in the earthenware, securing, so they said in 1886, 'the maximum of cleanliness'. Morrison, Ingram and Co. introduced a similar delivery arrangement in 1883 which they called the 'noiseless and steamless' system, claiming that it was less noisy than conventional taps and that it lessened the tendency of the hot water to evaporate and throw steam into the room.[44] Some baths and basins were filled at low level through a combination cock where the hot and cold water was mixed entering the bath or basin through just one inlet. But ultimately these systems were discredited because there was a risk of mains water being contaminated by foul water and soap that could be sucked through the low-level combination cock and syphoned into the supply pipes.[45]

Basins were also sometimes fitted with a shampoo apparatus. Shampoo referred not to the soap but to the actual washing of hair. The word was derived from the Hindu word 'champna', to squeeze

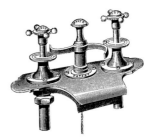

Interlocking bath or lavatory valves designed to prevent the waste of water, *c.* 1889. The taps could not be opened at the same time as the waste as they were locked by the catch fixed to the handle of the waste in the centre. The taps had cross handles and printed china discs and were set into a large plate with a mouth or inlet overhanging the edge of the bath. The unit was finished in lacquered brass.

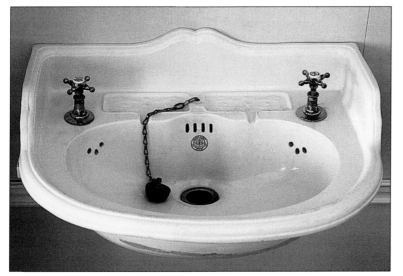

Shanks's 'Citizen' washbasin, *c.* 1890, with inlets in the side of the bowl.

and became widely used towards the end of the nineteenth century for the washing of hair. The London firm, Spong and Co., best known for their mincing machines, advertised a portable shampoo device in about 1895 and stated, 'shampooing at home is a necessity as well as a luxury. For health and cleanliness it is invaluable and is recommended strongly by the medical faculty.'[46] Shampoo devices varied: some consisted of an ascending spray, others of a long, swan-necked pipe or flexible rubber tube with a small shower rose on the end that received the hot and cold water mixed through a combination cock.

The waste pipes for draining the used water from the fitting were stopped with brass plugs on chains, although by the mid-1890s rubber plugs were coming into use. Some chains were weighted to draw the plug up against the top of the slab, 'preventing the annoyance of picking it out of the basin where it frequently falls . . . stopping the free discharge of the water'.[47] Wastes were also regulated by valves controlled from a pull-up knob which was often combined in a brass casting with the inlet valves. In Shanks's 'Patent Combined Bath' of 1886, for example, the hot and cold taps and the lift-up waste knob were fixed to a shelf cast in the end of the bath that was covered with a porcelain plate containing soap trays that drained into the waste.[48] In the mid-1890s, Doulton produced a

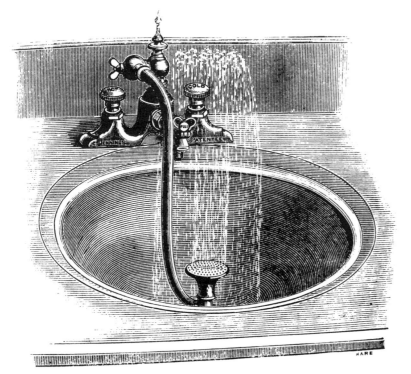

Patent shampooing shower and spray apparatus by George Jennings, Stangate, London. 'By raising and reversing the swan neck a shower is obtained for the head and neck, most agreeable and refreshing in hot climates.' *Martineau and Smith's Hardware Trade Journal*, 29 April 1882. (*Rural History Centre*)

range of five decorated porcelain bath trays for either parallel or taper baths. Overflow outlets were made to carry away any excess water through careless users leaving the taps running. Some were badly designed being connected directly to the soil pipe, bypassing the outlet trap and allowing sewer gas to reach the bath, but combined waste and overflow arrangements were standard among the leading manufacturers by the 1880s. They were securely trapped with either an S, or turn-down trap or the P, the shoot-out trap placed as near as possible to the underside of the bath or basin.

Late Victorian bathrooms were furnished with a range of accessories. Towel rails for fixing to walls or hot-water rails either polished brass or nickel-plated had appeared by the 1890s. Ornate holders, which could be screwed to the wall beside the washstand, were made to hold soap, sponges, toothbrushes and toothbrush powder. Bath racks for soap and sponges designed to bridge the top of the bath or hook onto the rim were introduced, and the 1900 catalogue of F.W. Webb of Boston even included wall-mounted cigar rests and match holders. Bath mats were laid on the floor and where gas was laid on a lamp bracket was often fitted beside the washbasin. But what of the third principal component, the water closet? Although the sanitary ideal was to install the water closet in a separate room it often formed part of the bathroom, and by the 1890s could be had *en suite* with the other fittings. Some of the most dramatic and impressive of those 'rapid strides' remarked upon by *The Ironmonger* in 1886 concerned the water closet.

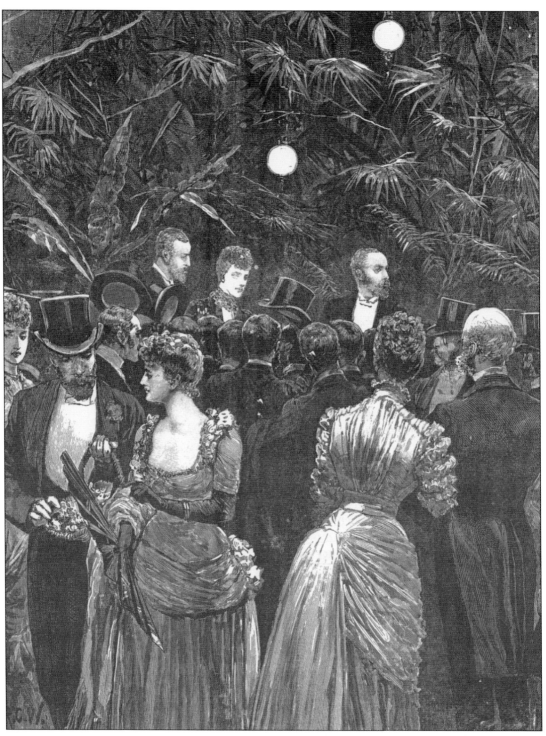

An evening fête for the benefit of the London hospitals at the International Health Exhibition, July 1884. Many prominent sanitaryware manufacturers were represented, including the firm George Jennings which exhibited their latest design, the 'Pedestal Vase' wash-out closet – one of the very first all-ceramic, free-standing water closets to have a pedestal base which enclosed the water-sealed trap. *Illustrated London News,* 2 August 1884

CHAPTER SEVEN

Absolute Perfection!
the development of the pedestal water closet

Fireworks exploded in the balmy night air. Chinese lanterns suspended from trees lit the faces of the fashionably dressed crowds who had flocked to the scene. It was the summer of 1884 and this was one of the evening soirées staged at the International Health Exhibition in South Kensington. Probably few of those watching the fireworks gave much thought to the important issues presented in the exhibition: public health, sanitation and personal hygiene. Britain and its people were cleaner than ever before and much of the sanitary-ware that had brought this about was on display in the exhibition. But within the galleries, an entirely new device was making its debut – the all-ceramic, free-standing water closet with a pedestal base which enclosed the unsightly bend of the water-sealed trap.

Following the introduction of valve and pan closets in the late eighteenth century, few improvements of any significance were made to water closets until the 1850s and 1860s. Valve and pan closets continued to be fixed inside wooden cabinets, while cheaper hopper and cottage closets were embedded in plinths of brick, rubble and mortar. With their fixed seats and round holes, water closets of every variety looked little different on the outside from the basic privy. Then from the 1870s, the pace of development quickened, and within a hectic twenty years, from about 1875, the water closet was changed beyond all recognition. But such was the pace of change that some of the new types were themselves swiftly rendered obsolete, condemned by sanitarians and overtaken by other innovations. The evolution of the water closet in these years, therefore, was anything but straightforward, and it is impossible to attribute the 'invention' of the modern, all-ceramic water closet to any one individual. It was rather a case that its development was muddled and uncertain, with rival manufacturers attempting to carve a niche in the market with their own particular design. During the late 1870s and 1880s, no single idea predominated and water-closet development progressed simultaneously along several lines. And then suddenly the confusion was over. By the early 1890s, the majority of manufacturers and leading sanitarians had come down in favour of the wash-down closet which was to become the standard British 'loo' of the twentieth century.

As towns and cities gradually adopted the water-carriage system for the removal of sewage, the water closet increasingly became a common fixture in British homes. But some of the impetus for its development after 1850 came from the need to provide facilities for public use in buildings such as hospitals, schools and railway stations. At precisely the mid-point of the century, in 1851, George Jennings secured a contract to supply the public conveniences in the three refreshment rooms at the Great Exhibition in Hyde Park. A charge was made for the use of some facilities and when the exhibition closed, receipts from these totalled £2,441.[1] The principle of paying to use public water closets was established, and a new toilet euphemism was born: 'to spend a penny'.[2] About a dozen manufacturers had water closets on display in the exhibition – but it was Jennings's closets providing a public service which offered a clue to the future.[3]

Jennings chose his 'india-rubber tube' valve closet for the 'superior' refreshment court but some of the closets he installed were of an entirely new design.[4] Like the hopper or cottage closet, this was an all-ceramic device – there were no valves – and the basin and trap were made in one piece. The interior, therefore, was completely free of joints, and in this respect alone it marked an important step in the development of the all-ceramic closet. It was also unusual in containing a wide, shallow pool of water held behind a weir or lip in the bowl separate from the water in the trap below. The idea was clearly to combine the simplicity of the hopper pan with the large surface area of water found in the typical valve closet. Valves, of course, were not suitable for closets likely to be subjected to rough and heavy use by the public, so Jennings opted for the water-sealed trap used on hopper pans. But hopper closets were also unsuited to heavy use: lacking an adequate pool of water to absorb the waste, filth accumulated inside the pan which was then difficult to remove. So, by providing two levels of water, Jennings created a closet that would immerse the solids, while providing a simple and effective seal from the soil pipe. The outlet and flush inlet were placed at the back, and when the flush water reached the shallow basin it forced the foul water over a weir into the trap below.

Jennings later claimed to have devised this closet before the exhibition, although it was only patented in 1852.[5] It went by various names – the Jennings basin, the 'monkey' closet and the

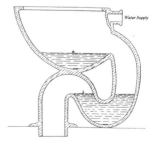

Jennings's valveless closet of 1852, as illustrated in his patent. This type of pan was developed as the wash-out closet from the mid-1870s.

Josiah George Jennings (1810–82)

EORGE JENNINGS was born at Totton, Southampton on 11 November 1810. He had no formal apprenticeship, but worked with his uncle who was a plumber and glazier. He moved to London in 1831 and set up on his own in Lambeth and then in 1838 at Charlotte Street, Blackfriars. In 1857 he moved to Holland Street, Blackfriars and finally to Palace Wharf, Stangate, where, by the 1890s, the company employed over 1,000 men.

George Jennings was unquestionably one of the greatest sanitary pioneers of Victorian Britain. He displayed considerable technical ingenuity and was responsible for many important innovations between the 1850s and the 1870s. Not all his ideas were a success, but he can be credited with the invention of wash-out closets, twin basin or plug closets, valveless water waste preventers and tip-up wash-basins. His first patent, for india-rubber lined taps, was taken out in 1847, and for this he was presented with a Royal Society of Arts medal in person by Prince Albert. In 1851 he offered to install the public conveniences at the Great Exhibition. His offer was initially turned down, but eventually accepted and he was awarded a prize for his water closet. The success of his facilities led to similar contracts at many important international trade fairs, including London in 1862, Paris in 1867 and Philadelphia in 1876, ensuring worldwide recognition for his sanitary fittings. He also constructed the sanitary fittings at the British hospitals at Varna and Scutari during the Crimean War.

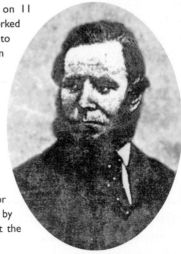

George Jennings. (*Russell-Cotes Art Gallery and Museum*)

In his early patents Jennings described himself as a brass founder, but he subsequently became involved in other manufactures relating to the production of sanitaryware. In 1854 he founded the South Western Pottery at Parkstone, Poole, Dorset. This became famous for its manufacture of sanitaryware and his own patent drain pipes as well as chimney pots, decorative brickwork and terracotta. His stoneware drain pipes were used for the laying of main drains in Portsmouth. Appreciating the value of india-rubber as a sealant in sanitaryware, he began his own production of rubber goods in London and at a branch factory in Birmingham. His forty or so patents included an improved rubber band and several varieties of seals for bottles and jars. His other business ventures included the development of housing in Clapham near his home.

He died on 17 April 1882 following a carriage accident and was buried at Norwood Cemetery, London. He married twice and had fifteen children and after his death the business was carried on by his sons who continued to use his name. They introduced one of the very first pedestal water closets, the 'Pedestal Vase' in 1884, and then in 1894, 'The Closet of the Century', one of the best-known British syphonic closets.

'complete' closet (because it combined pan, trap and soil pipe in one piece); in the 1870s, when further development of the type took place, it became known as the 'wash-out' or 'flush-out' closet. Surprisingly, perhaps, Jennings played little or no part in this future development. Instead, he turned to improving valve closets, which, at the time went unchallenged for what the plumbers called 'good quality work'. In 1856, he patented the addition of rubber rings to the valve and its seating.[6] Then, two years later, he turned to the development of closets discharged by operating a plunger or piston in place of the conventional rotating valve. Jennings added a vertical cylinder or secondary basin at the back of the closet that contained a

plug and vertical rod in an elastic seating. When the plug was raised
by a pull of the handle, the flush water was simultaneously released,
washing the contents of the basin through the connection to the rear
basin and then through the open outlet.[7] In 1863 John Shanks, then
a little-known plumber in Barrhead, near Glasgow, patented a
similar device with an india-rubber ball serving as the plug. The
closet basin was connected by a short inclined pipe to a separate
cylinder containing the plug: there was no trap, the flexible rubber
ball providing the necessary seal from the soil pipe. Another feature
of the closet was the fitting of a cistern with a ball cock to one side of
the cylinder behind the basin. This was Shanks's first patent – many
more were to follow – but at the time his premises consisted of
nothing more than a makeshift brass foundry above a plumber's shop
in a converted saw pit. Shanks obtained his cast-iron parts from
George Smith and Co. of the Sun Foundry, Glasgow and his
earthenware closet basins from J.M.P. Bell in Glasgow.[8]

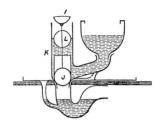

Section of Shanks's Patent
Flexible Valve Closet, his
'Number Four', patented in
1863. The drawing shows the
india-rubber plug, J, and the
ballcock regulating the water
level in the cistern, L.

Shanks named his closet the 'Patent Flexible Valve Closet' (catchy
trade names still lay in the future), although in the works it was
simply known by its catalogue number, the 'Number Four'. It
brought success to John Shanks and formed the basis of the firm's
subsequent expansion. According to his nephew, William, 'it had a
great vogue all over the country'.[9] When the Prince of Wales fell
dangerously ill with typhoid at Sandringham in November 1871,
investigations at the royal residences revealed that at Buckingham
Palace every sanitary device was defective except the Shanks
'Number Four' in the servants' quarters.[10] Upon his recovery, the
prince was sufficiently impressed to pronounce that had he not been
born a prince he would have been a plumber. The chief attraction of
the closet was its relative simplicity: an advertisement of the early
1870s for the 'Number Four' emphasised its 'durability, facility of
erection and cheapness'.[11]

George Jennings's twin-basin
closet made in one piece of
earthenware, on the left,
illustrated in Thomas
Twyford's catalogue published
in March 1879. These closets
were also made in two parts
with the plug cylinder and
trap in galvanised iron. By
1894 upwards of 128,000 of
these side-outlet closets had
been sold since their
introduction in the 1860s,
although in 1890 the company
modified the design and
removed the plug chamber
which, by then, was widely
condemned as insanitary.

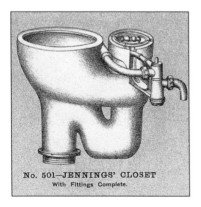

No. 501–JENNINGS' CLOSET
With Fittings Complete.

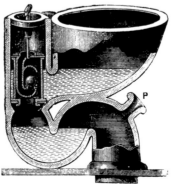

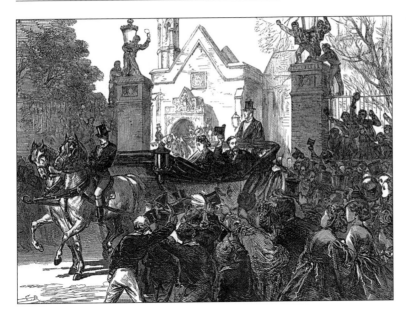

The Prince of Wales leaves Sandringham for Windsor after his recovery from typhoid in February 1872. *Illustrated London News,* 17 February 1872

Jennings, meanwhile, must have been sufficiently encouraged by sales of his own plug closet to make further improvements. In 1866 he altered the design of the discharge valve to a hollow piston which acted as an overflow from the basin to the trap. Jennings, unlike Shanks, retained a water-sealed trap and had some made entirely of earthenware.[12] In 1878 he supplied 550 of his patent valve closets and trap in one piece to the massive Palace Hotel in San Francisco, which, at the time, claimed to surpass in grandeur all the hotels of Europe and America.[13] In the 1870s they were also made by Thomas Twyford in Hanley and were included in the Twyford catalogue for 1879. For a while, the future looked promising for trapless and twin-basin closets. By 1881 Jennings claimed to have sold 'upwards of 50,000' of his patent valve closet and trap since its introduction; he also introduced a trapless version, suitable for use with well-ventilated soil pipes. In 1875, J. Bailey Denton commended Jennings's twin basin for 'its simplicity of construction and compactness'. However, he added that it would be better if provided with a trapped overflow from the pan, instead of relying on the hollow plug, which, he explained, 'will allow effluvia generated in the trap to pass through the plug into the closet'.[14] This was the obvious problem with twin-basin closets: foul water could pass freely from the front pan to the cylinder with its piston or plug. S. Stevens Hellyer was more critical still, roundly condemning the trapless variety for its tendency to pass sewer gas into the room every time it was flushed, and again emphasised the weakness of the hollow valve which could leak foul water and fumes. But as late as 1884, *The Ironmonger* carried an advertisement for Pearson's patent

'Twin Basin' closet made of one piece of earthenware. Patented in 1874, it was made by Capper and Son of Fenchurch Street, London (not to be confused with Thomas Crapper) who claimed that it had been used at Guy's Hospital since about 1875.[15] By the mid-1880s, however, other important developments in water-closet design were under way, and in the 1890s the development of trapless and twin-basin closets ground to a halt. Hellyer delivered the final blow in 1891 when he said, 'no sanitarian of authority would allow such a closet to be fixed on any of his works'.[16]

'In a number of cases where these [Shanks's 'Number 4' closets] have been fitted up, I have felt a bad smell come up through the overflow of the cistern.'
William Buchan, Glasgow, 1876.

S. Stevens Hellyer was indisputably an influential sanitarian of the late nineteenth century. His most famous publication, *The Plumber and Sanitary Houses*, first published in 1877, eventually ran to six editions and was even translated into French.[17] But he was also a sanitaryware manufacturer and hardly, therefore, a disinterested observer. Perhaps it was no coincidence that he had taken out a patent the previous year for a water closet similar to Jennings's all-ceramic pan of the early 1850s with its two levels of water and no valves, cranks or levers. There had been little apparent interest in closets of this type following Jennings's patent in 1852. The distinctive profile of this closet appears in two patents of the 1860s, but it was not until the mid-1870s that further development occurred when, within a short period of time, several leading sanitaryware manufacturers patented improvements to Jennings's original design.[18]

Hellyer promoted the wash-out in his book and even took the credit for the invention himself – one can only imagine, to Jennings's surprise and irritation.[19] This water closet, he explained, 'was invented by the writer but patented by Mr Rowley . . . to whom it was entrusted to be made'. Samuel Hunt Rowley was a potter in Swadlincote, south Derbyshire, where ceramic sanitaryware had been manufactured since the mid-nineteenth century. Having received an order from Hellyer to make an improved version of Jennings's closet, Rowley promptly made it the subject of his own patent in February 1875. Rowley kept the outlet at the back, as in Jennings's original design, but moved the inlet around to the front. This greatly improved the flushing capability of the pan. Now the waste was pushed over the lip or weir by the full force of the flush into the trap below. Rowley also diverted a small portion of the flush to a perforated pipe that cleaned the sides of the basin.[20] In March 1878 Rowley's partner in Swadlincote, James Woodward, registered the name 'Wash-out' as a trade name for the closet. Of course, this did not stop other manufacturers using the name, but whenever wash-out closets, in general, were recommended, Woodward and Rowley were able to take all the credit, as well as informing the public that theirs was the only genuine article. This time, it was probably the turn of Hellyer – the joint employer of the largest firm of plumbers in the country – to feel aggrieved![21]

Hellyer's 1876 patent for a wash-out closet specified a pan made with, 'an outlet arranged at the front so as to be concealed by the seat'.[22] 'The outlet at the back', he explained, 'where everything is exposed to view is somewhat objectionable.'[23] Even on this detail, Hellyer was not first: John Dodd, a Liverpool sanitaryware manufacturer, had patented one with a flushing rim and front outlet shortly after Rowley in 1875. Then in 1877 Daniel Bostel, a Brighton sanitary engineer, patented another with a front outlet made with a removable cover so that, using a plunger, the vertical passage of the outlet could be cleared of obstructions.[24] Other new wash-out closets quickly followed. John Dodd took out a second patent for one in August 1878,[25] and in March 1879 Thomas Twyford published a new catalogue that featured his first wash-out closet, the 'National', made in one piece of earthenware with the outlet placed at the side. Doulton and Co. had also introduced their 'Lambeth' wash-out closet by 1879.

The revival of the wash-out principle from the mid-1870s marked the growing importance of the sanitaryware potter in water-closet design. Most wash-out closets were made entirely of earthenware (although some had metal traps) and most of the makers involved in their development from 1875 were potters, such as Woodward and Rowley, Doulton, Twyford and the original maker, George Jennings, who had established a pottery in Poole, Dorset in 1854. Writing in about 1898, Joseph Hatton, Twyford's own historian, recalled how, in the 1870s, Thomas Twyford developed the 'National' as an all-ceramic closet, frustrated that his firm received just 2s for the earthenware basin of a pan closet, while the brass and iron founder made from 20s to 50s. It is unlikely that he was the only potter who resented the unequal share of the profits, and this may have been behind Samuel Hunt Rowley's decision to take out patent protection in 1875.

Although the wash-out was well received by sanitary experts, the manufacturers, however, came up against a commonly encountered barrier: the innate conservatism of the consumer. At first, sales of Twyford's 'National' were poor, just 50 were sold during the first year of its production and only about 200 the following year.[26] All-ceramic water closets in the form of hopper and cottage basins had been around for a long time, but they were inclined to smell and, moreover, were associated with servants and the working classes. There was a strong supposition that a good-quality water closet had

'Plug closets, however, with or without a trap are not necessarily satisfactory.'

Shirley Foster Murphy, 1883.

to have a valve, in addition to a water-sealed trap, to create a second barrier against sewer gas in the soil pipe. For most of the nineteenth century, the miasma theory, which held that disease was carried in foul air, remained current. Smells, therefore, were not only offensive but potentially dangerous. Even if the closet was trapless, like Shanks's 'Number Four', the inclusion of some mechanics probably helped fill the middle-class customer with confidence. It took several years of support from leading sanitary engineers and doctors before the public was finally convinced that the wash-out was reliable – and respectable.

By the early 1880s, public confidence in the wash-out closet was growing and sales of Twyford's 'National' were soon reaching 10,000 a year. In 1882, he introduced a second model, the 'Crown', a cheaper version with a separate basin and trap.[27] While the earthenware 'National' could be had with coloured decoration or with an ivy pattern, the 'Crown' was made of fireclay with the cane or yellow-coloured exterior, typical of hopper and other cheap closets, and a white-glazed interior. Twyford promoted the 'Crown' for use in factories, barracks and other places where 'a large number of persons are employed and where a good strong closet basin is necessary'.[28] In 1883, they introduced a third wash-out model, the 'Alliance', which was similar to the 'National' but with the outlet placed at the front and hidden from view by the seat. By the mid-1880s, wash-out closets were being made by sanitaryware potters across the country: Sharpe Brothers in Swadlincote, the Crown Clay Co. in Bristol[29] and Joseph Cliff and Sons of Wortley, Leeds. Potters also made the ceramic fittings for other sanitaryware companies such as Shanks, Morrison, Ingram and Co. in Manchester, Charles Winn and Co. of Birmingham and Thomas Crapper who obtained his ceramicware from among others, Twyfords and Sharpe Brothers in Swadlincote.

From the late 1870s, new models were usually distinguished by snappy trade names designed to impress and beguile the public. Encouraged by trademark legislation introduced in 1875 and 1876, the names varied from the grandiose to the mundane: some suggested a royal connection, like Twyford's 'Crown,' while others were drawn from the factory site, such as Shanks's 'Tubal' and Frederick Humpherson's 'Beaufort'. Some of the names drew attention to a particular feature of the device, such as Jennings's 'Deep Seal' and quite a few, like the 'Deluge' and 'Torrent' hinted at the effectiveness of the flushing action. Some were made by joining together the factory name with a local place or even the name of a senior company man: thus was created the 'Twycliffe' and the 'Sharcote', shorthand for Sharpe's of Swadlincote, but sometimes, as with the 'Kenon' and the 'Spedan', the names are not so easily decoded.

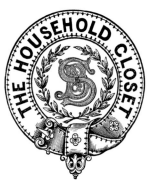

Underglaze transfer printed maker's mark from a wash-down closet of 1895 by Sharpe Brothers, Swadlincote, Derbyshire. (*Sharpe Bros and Co. Ltd, Swadlincote*)

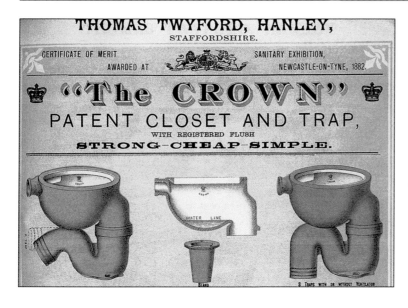

THOMAS TWYFORD, HANLEY,
STAFFORDSHIRE.

CERTIFICATE OF MERIT
AWARDED AT

SANITARY EXHIBITION,
NEWCASTLE-ON-TYNE, 1882.

✠ "The CROWN" ✠
PATENT CLOSET AND TRAP,
WITH REGISTERED FLUSH
STRONG—CHEAP—SIMPLE.

'The Crown', Twyford's cheapest wash-out closet in cane and white fireclay, from their 1883 catalogue. The outlet was at the side so the bowl required a separate stand which is seen here to support the underside of the pan. Wash-out closets like this were usually enclosed in a wooden cabinet. (*Twyford Bathrooms*)

This was a vital period for the development of the water closet. Public interest in sanitary science had never been greater: the volume of literature available on the subject increased and in the 1870s exhibitions of sanitaryware were arranged by the Royal Society of Arts, the Social Science Association and the Royal Sanitary Institute, founded in 1876. The first exhibition organised by the Sanitary Institute was held in Stafford in 1878, and in subsequent years their autumn congress became an important annual event for the industry. The exhibition stands enabled manufacturers to promote their latest models, while prominent sanitary engineers, architects and medical doctors were invited to give papers on matters of public health, plumbing techniques and sanitary fittings. The meetings reflected current thinking and new trends: an early casualty was the pan closet that was roundly condemned by sanitarians such as William Eassie, while the wash-out closet clearly benefited from all the extra exposure. At the institute's meeting in 1879, held at Croydon, Daniel Bostel exhibited his wash-out closet, the 'Brighton Excelsior', Beard, Dent and Hellyer were also there with their 'Vortex' model, while Doulton and Co. exhibited their version of the wash-out, the 'Lambeth' (along with, of course, some of their art pottery).[30] Exhibits which caught the attention of expert judges were awarded prize medals or certificates of merit which the makers then capitalised on in their advertising. Twyford's 1883 catalogue, for example, highlighted the fact that the 'National' wash-out closet had collected awards in South Kensington and Brighton in 1881 and Newcastle in 1882.[31] Sanitation also reached the national press. In a letter to the *Daily Telegraph* in September 1880, a medical officer of health stated that 'The Local Government Board forbids the use of these pan closets . . . they may be easily replaced by one of the wash-out closet basins.'[32] Sanitation was suddenly topical – and fashionable.

In the summer of 1884 the largest show of all, the International Health Exhibition, was held in the grounds of the Royal Horticultural Society in South Kensington. With the Prince of Wales as president this vast exhibition, known at the time as the 'Healtheries', occupied a 30-acre covered space and was a major national event visited by 4.2 million people. Although many of the displays had little to do with sanitation and many people were drawn by the promise of the nocturnal fêtes – not displays of closet pans and drainpipes – an entire gallery was dedicated to bathroom and sanitary equipment. Two houses were erected in the grounds showing the worst and best practice in drainage and sanitation. Many prominent names in the sanitaryware trade attended, including Doulton, Jennings, Twyford and Shanks, presenting the latest ideas in all-ceramic free-standing water closets.[33]

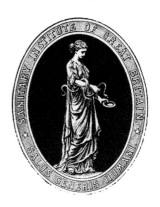

The Greek goddess, Hygeia, was chosen as the emblem for the Royal Sanitary Institute of Great Britain, founded in 1876.

The growing popularity of the wash-out had everything to do with its performance and nothing to do with its looks. Whether made in one or two pieces of earthenware, early wash-outs were awkward and ungainly. Versions with a side outlet usually required additional support under the basin, while those with a front or side outlet had an ugly projecting nose or trunk. Most early wash-outs, therefore, continued to be enclosed within a wooden bench that contained the traditional lift-up handle to operate the flush. But in this period of rapid development, every aspect of closet design came under scrutiny: if the interior could be streamlined by removing plugs, pans and valves, then it just remained to simplify the exterior – to do away with the old wooden cabinet – and produce a completely sanitary device. From the early 1880s, makers developed closets that could stand without an enclosure. By 1883 Shanks had introduced an 'encased washing out closet' in which the earthenware basin and trap were enclosed in an iron shell or case filled with concrete.[34] In January 1884 Shanks claimed to have sold 'many hundreds' to hospitals and to private customers, but this device did not remain in Shanks's catalogues for long. The answer lay in making all-ceramic pedestal closets, and inevitably sanitaryware potters took the lead in their development.

'It would go far to promote cleanliness and prevent this smell if the seat enclosure was entirely dispensed with.' Shirley Foster Murphy, 1883.

One of the very first was the 'Pedestal Vase' made by George Jennings and Co. According to a review of the International Health Exhibition in *The Builder*, George Jennings showed 'his new "Pedestal Vase" wash-out closet with trap inside the pedestal, which stands well clear of the wall at back and sides and needs no boxing in at the front'.[35] Doulton exhibited their 'Combination' wash-out closet in the exhibition. This was a wash-out basin and trap of decorated stoneware designed to stand without an enclosure; it was still a two-piece closet with an exposed trap, but it soon reappeared as a sinuous all-in-one closet with the trap enclosed within the pedestal.[36] In 1886 Shanks's 'Tubal' wash-out – which was also displayed at South Kensington in 1884 – was illustrated as a fully enclosed pedestal closet. Twyford soon launched his own version of the pedestal closet, the 'Unitas'.

Thomas Twyford began development of his first free-standing closet, the 'Unitas', in about 1884. The first examples were made with a separate trap that was still exposed, but the overall shape was more compact and attractive than that of the 'National' or 'Crown'. The front outlet was straight-sided and did not project beyond the rim of the basin and, as if to emphasise that this all-ceramic device was fit to be seen, the exterior was moulded with a relief design of oak leaves and acorns. In early 1885 the 'Unitas' was praised in the journal *Building News* for its high degree of 'cleanliness, utility and simplicity'. According to Hatton, the impetus for further development of the 'Unitas' came that summer when the firm's agent in Paris received an enquiry from an architect who asked if Twyfords could supply a closet that was 'fixed open and exposed without any wood enclosure'. Working with some of his most experienced potters in Hanley, Twyford produced a large and complicated piece of pottery in which the basin and trap were enclosed within a sleek exterior casing. In Paris the architect was so pleased with the result that he ordered 700 for the large apartments he was building there.[37]

At last the water closet was made a thing of beauty. The 'Unitas' was available in plain ivory or white earthenware and also in cane and white fireclay, but more expensive models were made with the oak design in relief around the front and sides of the pedestal. In 1886 Twyfords added a new raised pattern, 'Florentine', which complemented the fashion among the better-off for the Renaissance style in their bathrooms.[38] Both these designs could be had in plain white, ivory or colour,

The 'Pedestal Vase', probably the first pedestal water closet to make a public appearance, at the International Health Exhibition in May 1884, where it was awarded a gold medal. The closet had a wash-out pan with a front outlet and was made in one piece of 'highly glazed porcelain'. In an official test at the exhibition the closet was coupled to a 2-gallon syphonic cistern and successfully disposed of ten apples, a flat sponge and four pieces of sanitary paper stuck to the sides with plumbers' smudge. (*Thomas Crapper and Co. Ltd*)

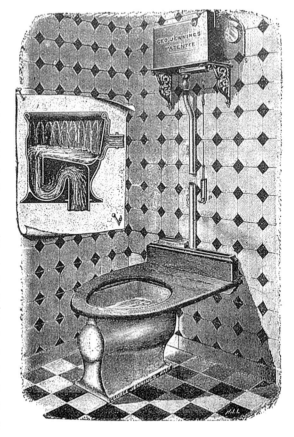

inside and out. The attention to detail, however, did not stop at the pedestal and bowl. The mahogany seat was supported by cast-iron brackets which incorporated the word 'Unitas' within the ornate scrollwork, and at the back of the seat there was a decorative ceramic paper box complementing the style of the pedestal. The cast-iron cistern was painted to match the inlet pipe and seat brackets and was operated by a pendant pull and chain which was neatly held in place by an ebonised block with brass fittings.

The pedestal offered ambitious potters endless opportunities to experiment with form and decoration. The front outlet, which had become general on wash-out closets by the mid-1880s, imposed what was known in the trade as the 'full front' pedestal. While Twyford covered theirs with oak leaves or Renaissance-inspired scrollwork, Shanks went for a somewhat formal 'architectural' (their word) design. Then in December 1884 J. Dimmock and Co. of the Albion Works, Hanley, introduced one of the most celebrated designs of all time, the 'Dolphin'.[39] This magnificent creation took the form of a dolphin-headed sea serpent with open jaws holding a giant shell which formed the pan. The S or shoot-down trap was a continuation of the body of the creature. In

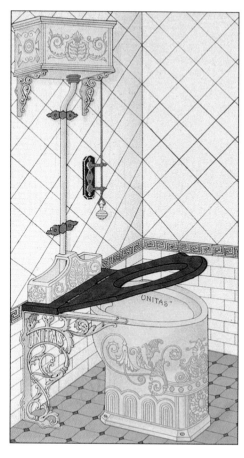

September 1886 Joseph Cliff and Sons, of Wortley, near Leeds, who owned Dimmock and Co., exhibited the 'Dolphin' at the Sanitary Institute's congress at York. A reviewer of the exhibition, writing in *The Builder* was impressed: 'even in garish white and gold, it is perhaps preferable to the ivy clad tree stump-like pedestals which are being used for closets of this kind.'[40] Another zoomorphic design was Baxendale's 'Lion' closet, introduced in 1886, which had a pan resting on the back of a recumbent lion.[41] Also in 1886 the London manufacturers, Smeaton and Sons, patented a hopper closet enclosed in a pedestal which was available in two shapes, one based on a classical amphora and the other on a sea creature, the nautilus.[42] The pedestal enclosure, therefore, was not restricted solely to wash-out basins. The novel modelling of Smeaton's pedestal also attracted praise, this time from *The Ironmonger*, which, in 1892, reported 'the elegance of the design cannot fail to give it a leading position among the sanitary appliances of the day'.[43] Jockeying for pole position in sales was behind this sudden burst of creative closet design: exterior styling was second only to the practical efficiency of the appliance. The result was a vast range of models for the consumer to choose

Twyford's 'Unitas' – one of the finest pedestal wash-out closets of the 1880s. The trap is enclosed by the ceramic pedestal, which in the more expensive models was covered with relief decoration. Twyford's were early pioneers of this with their oak-leaf design introduced in about 1884. This one is in the 'Florentine' pattern introduced in 1886 in ivory with matching paper box and cistern. The closet has a mahogany lifting seat supported on galvanised brackets and a pendant pull held in an ebony block. (*Twyford Bathrooms*)

from and in some instances, the creation of closets of sensational beauty.

Pedestal closets may have been eye-catching, but they also accorded with the latest ideas on sanitary hygiene. While the miasma theory still attracted influential support – notably from Edwin Chadwick and Florence Nightingale – medical research had established beyond all doubt the connection between germs and dirt. From the 1880s germ theory led to an increased awareness of the importance of personal hygiene and frequent domestic cleaning. At the International Health Exhibition, Jennings's 'Pedestal Vase' closet attracted favourable comment from *The Builder* for the ease with which the floor surrounding the closet could be 'readily cleansed with mop or house flannel'. The boxing-in of the closet, which for so long had been the norm, was now condemned as insanitary. The wooden casing could harbour dust and dirt and even vermin. In 1886, *The Health Journal* likened the wooden cabinet to a dustbin – 'an abomination in cases where servants are not very systematic in the removal of rubbish'.[44] The condemnation of wooden enclosures also affected bath and washbasin design, and although grandiose wood panelling remained popular for more than a decade for those who could afford it, the latest ideas on sanitary hygiene and germ theory demanded free-standing appliances.

'The Dolphin . . . represents not only the perfection of cleanliness but is an ornament to any bathroom. It is efficient in operation and without any moving or mechanical parts liable to get out of order. The Dolphin is made in England and guaranteed not to craze or discolour.'
J.L. Mott Ironworks, New York and Chicago.

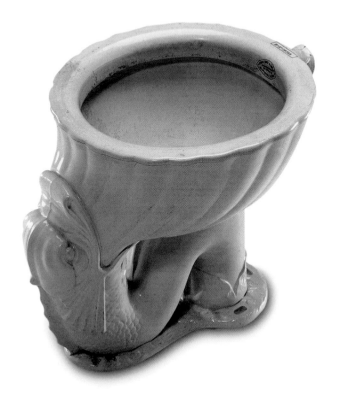

An ivory 'Dolphin' wash-out closet, a design registered by J. Dimmock and Co. of Hanley on 31 December 1884. The company was owned by Joseph Cliff and Sons, fireclay manufacturers in Wortley, Leeds. The Dolphin was also available highlighted in blue and even gold lustre. This particular one is stamped 'Cliff' and was sold by Stock, Sons and Taylor of Birmingham. (*Thomas Crapper and Co. Ltd*)

The adoption of the lifting seat with the pedestal closet also contributed, in the view of many, to making a cleaner and more versatile device. Several closets on display at the International Health Exhibition were provided with a lifting seat, exposing what was described as an 'earthenware slop top' when it was raised. This enabled the closet to be used as a urinal and sink for slops; the combination of these functions was the inspiration behind Doulton's choice of 'Combination' as the name for their pedestal wash-out closet.[45] Of course, the old cabinet closets with fixed seats had been used as urinals and for slopping out chamber pots, but with unpleasant consequences. As Twyford pointed out in an 1888 advertisement for the 'Unitas', lifting the hinged seat allowed the closet to be used as a urinal, without 'the "wetting" so objectionable in closets having permanent seats'.[46] But not everyone was convinced this was a healthy development. In 1891 Hellyer wrote, 'as it has now become the bad practice with many men to treat such closets as if they were urinals, it will generally be found that there is more filth outside such closets than inside'.[47] Doubtless, some of Hellyer's readers – women especially – would have agreed with him, and ever since the lift-up seat was introduced in the 1880s, women have had to contend with another irritation: finding the seat left up by the last careless male user.

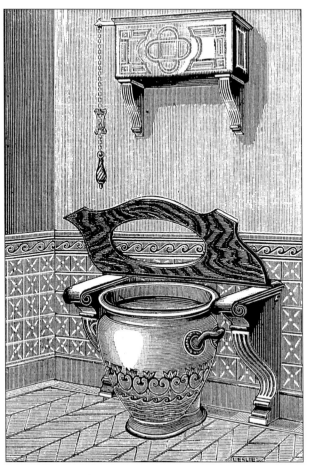

One of the more distinctive pedestal closets of the 1880s was the 'Amphora' closet with a hopper bowl introduced by Smeaton and Sons, London, in 1886.

Nevertheless, the all-ceramic pedestal water closet was here to stay, but the world of sanitary science in the late nineteenth century was nothing if not fickle. No sooner had the wash-out closet reached near perfection as a multi-purpose, streamlined and often beautifully decorated appliance, doubts were raised about its effectiveness. It was again Hellyer who played a large part in marshalling the objections to the wash-out closet. The chief problem was that one flush of water had to clear two levels of water and generally, by the time the flush had shunted the foul water over the weir into the outlet, it had insufficient energy left to scour and clean the trap. The consequence, of course, was that the trap could harbour foul water which could smell. According to Hellyer, the excrement 'no matter', in his words, 'what state it has come from the body', is driven against the upper sides of the basin by the sudden inrush of water, leaving 'its marks' behind. At least this part of the device was visible and accessible and could be cleaned, but the large exposed surface between the weir and the water seal of the trap, which was not so accessible, could, over time, acquire a coating of 'faecal matter', which would also generate bad air. Another unpleasant feature of the typical wash-out closet in Hellyer's view was that the depth of water in the basin was insufficient to drown the solid waste. As he explained, this was a problem aggravated by 'a long seat holder' who would render the state of the atmosphere unbearable for some minutes to any other visitor.[48]

There was also a new water closet on the scene which, by the late 1880s, was attracting attention. This was the 'flush-down' or 'wash down' which took the development towards an even simpler basin and trap a step further. While the water-seal trap of a wash-out was placed some distance below the upper basin, in the wash-down it was actually within it. The exposed surface liable to be fouled was, therefore, considerably reduced, and in Hellyer's words, 'the force of the flush, instead of spending itself upon the basin as in the wash-out, passes through the trap with a scouring action, washing the whole of the interior'.[49] A greater security against sewer gas was also achieved through increasing the depth of water in the trap. The effectiveness of the wash-down was beyond all doubt and from the 1890s, it was swiftly established as the standard British water closet. But who was responsible for this important innovation?

The London firm of Humpherson and Co. is generally credited with introducing the wash-down closet. Their 'Beaufort' pedestal 'flush-down' water closet, named after their works in Chelsea, was exhibited at the 1885 Congress of the Sanitary Institute, Leicester and was awarded a Certificate of Merit. This was hardly a sensational debut: it was actually eclipsed by two dry privies at the show – one belonging to Moule's Earth Closet Co. and the other, Morrell's Sanitary Appliance Co., both, of which, came away with higher

'Twyford's Unitas . . . is not enclosed with wood work but is fully exposed so that no filth nor anything causing offensive smells can accumulate or escape detection.'
Thomas W. Twyford, 1887.

The 'Lillyman' basin and trap, a two-piece closet from Twyford's 1879 catalogue. The high level of water in the basin indicates that this was an early form of wash-down closet, although the term was not known at the time. This simple closet was also free standing as the trap is formed with a flanged foot that could be screwed to the floor. The 'Lillyman' was still on sale in 1894, by which time Twyford was describing it as a wash-down closet. (*Twyford Bathrooms*)

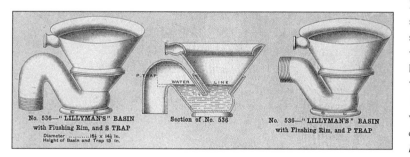

No. 536—"LILLYMAN'S" BASIN with Flushing Rim, and S TRAP
Diameter ....16½ × 14½ In.
Height of Basin and Trap 13 In.

Section of No. 536

No. 536—"LILLYMAN'S" BASIN with Flushing Rim, and P TRAP

awards. Doulton's 'Combination' wash-out closet was also given a
Certificate of Merit at Leicester.[50] The wash-out was then at the peak
of its popularity, and no one in 1885 seemed to doubt its
effectiveness; new models continued to appear for several years, and
for a while little was heard about the wash-down. But there was
another reason why Humpherson's 'Beaufort' probably raised so few
eyebrows: there really was nothing new about it, except the name.
The 'Beaufort' was essentially a short hopper or cottage closet with
the trap set higher, so the water line was within the basin – and these
had been around since the 1840s and 1850s.[51] Several patents taken
out between the 1850s and the 1870s feature hopper closets which
had the higher water level characteristic of the wash-down: for
example, a patent taken out on Christmas Eve 1879 by William
Buchan, a Glasgow sanitary engineer, shows a hopper closet that
could be made in one piece with a flanged base.[52] His specification
shows a high-water level inside the basin, or as he says 'on the closet
side of the trap', which he explained was 'widened in a conical form'
increasing the surface area of water in the bowl. This was a wash-
down closet in everything but name – as was Hellyer's 'Artisan'
which had appeared by 1877. This simple closet had a shallow basin
attached to a trap with a small flanged foot and again a good surface
area of water within the basin.[53] Twyford's 'Lillyman' basin and trap,
advertised in their catalogue of March 1879, was virtually
identical.[54]

The 'Beaufort' wash-down
closet was introduced in 1885
by Humpherson and Co.,
Chelsea. This was almost
certainly the first fully
enclosed pedestal wash-down
closet and the precursor of the
standard wash-down pedestal
'toilet' of the twentieth
century. This unadorned
example is in cane and
whiteware, but it was also
made with oak-leaf decoration
in relief around the outside of
the pedestal.

Thus the wash-down was not a new type of closet that suddenly
appeared in the mid-1880s as the successor to the wash-out. The fact
is, it had been around for just as long, only no one seems to have
realised that this simple and robust appliance was
equal if not superior to every other type of water
closet in use. Rudimentary pedestal versions had
appeared before 1880: it just needed someone to tidy
up the design and give the closet a new name to
distinguish it from the worst type of hopper and
cottage closets where the water level of the trap was
situated well below the basin. Frederick Humpherson
(1854–1919) did precisely this: as far as we know, the
name 'flush-down' was his; he produced in the
'Beaufort' a compact, effective and cheap closet that
was to have many imitators.

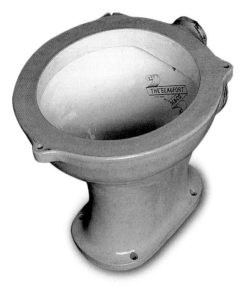

As an all-ceramic water closet, the wash-down
started life as a basic appliance supplied for the use of
servants and fitted in working-class homes. In 1877
Hellyer explained that he had designed the 'Artisan'
especially for artisans' dwellings where, he said, 'it

Frederick Humpherson (1854–1919)

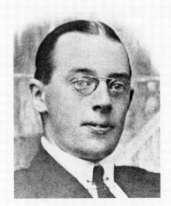

Frederick Humpherson.
(Original Bathrooms)

FREDERICK HUMPHERSON was the oldest son of Edward Humpherson from Chelsea, and in 1871 was apprenticed to Thomas Crapper. In 1876 Edward formed Humpherson and Co. with Frederick at 331 Kings Road, Chelsea. Their showrooms were at the end of nearby Beaufort Street and the corner of Fulham Road.

Frederick Humpherson took out four patents including one for a syphonic water-waste preventer in 1885 and another for a pedestal water closet in 1892. In 1885, when the free standing, all-ceramic pedestal closet was rapidly becoming fashionable for wash-out pans, Humpherson chose to use the pedestal form to enclose a basin and trap-type water closet. Humpherson called his closet the 'Beaufort' after his works, but also appears to have coined the term 'flush-down' or 'wash-down' as a general term for closets made with a water seal within the pan and not below it, as in hopper and cottage types. Simple two-piece closets were already in use, so Humpherson cannot be credited with the invention of the wash-down closet, but sanitarians and manufacturers clearly liked the name 'wash-down' and it was soon widely adopted. In this period of rapid development other makers soon had their own versions of the pedestal wash-down closet on the market. Nevertheless, Humpherson and Co. were able to claim, quite legitimately, that their 'Beaufort' was the 'original' pedestal wash-down closet.

When Humpherson died towards the end of 1919, he left the entire business to his younger brother, Alfred, who died in 1945, and in turn left the company to his son and daughter, Sydney and Edith. Edith's son Geoffrey Pidgeon entered the business in 1947 and sold the company in 1981, but immediately started Original Bathrooms (the name is taken from the original pedestal wash-down closet), based in Richmond, which is now run by Michael and John Pidgeon.

was important to have a simple and self-cleansing water closet . . . where a valve closet would be too expensive'.[55] By 1886, however, he could see the closet had wider appeal. In January that year, he claimed the 'Artisan' is 'so well known, and so extensively used, that hardly a word of explanation is needed'. He added, 'as the closet is fixed . . . largely for general purposes as for the use of mechanics and domestics and exception having been taken to the name "Artisan", it has been renamed the "Hygienic".'[56] Two surviving examples of Humpherson's 'Beaufort' are made of cane and white fireclay – the cheapest type of ceramicware used in water-closet manufacture. Twyfords first used the name 'wash-down' in 1887 when they introduced the 'Deluge' – not as a 'top of the range' model but as their cheapest item – cheaper, even, than the utilitarian 'Crown' wash-out closet. This first 'Deluge' was a two-piece closet in cane and white ware with an exposed trap and began life very much as a 'below stairs' – or servants' wing – appliance. The humble antecedents of the wash-down could not have been more apparent. Like Hellyer, Twyford soon appreciated that sales of wash-down closets need not be restricted to the lower end of the market. In 1889 it was relaunched as a handsome, fully enclosed, one piece ceramic pedestal closet similar to the 'Unitas': 'It has been improved,' Twyford announced, 'and its outside and general appearance, when made in one piece, approaches that of the 'Unitas.' As a one-piece article it was available in almost all the styles applied to the 'Unitas' – but not quite all. In 1889, the 'Unitas' was still Twyford's premier model, but the end of the wash-out closet was almost in sight.

By 1893, the 'Deluge' had been joined by the 'Cardinal' and both were available in a wide range of styles. Besides the basic white or ivory there were single-colour printed designs to choose from such as 'Mikado', 'Japanesque' or 'Poppy', and then there was the slightly more expensive multicoloured 'Chrysanthemum' or 'Azalea'. At the top of the range and costing twice as much again as any of these was the quite magnificent 'Venetian' pattern in raised ornament and coloured deep blue and gold. Even the cistern and paper box could be had to match. Twyford, of course, was not alone: Doulton and Co.

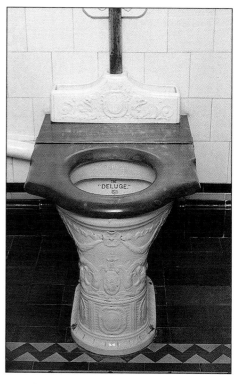

The 'Deluge' wash-down closet by Twyford's with raised decoration at Berwick House, near Shrewsbury, photographed in 1999, still in use with its original paper box and ceramic cistern after 100 years.

introduced their 'Simplicitas' wash-down closet and Shanks, the 'Citizen', which was available with their 'architectural' moulded ornament combined with hand-painted floral patterns in colour. Thomas Crapper introduced an improved 'Marlboro' wash-down, with an attractive decorative skirting hiding the trap, at about the same time. Johnson Brothers of Hanley launched the 'Latestas' in 1891 in polychrome floral decoration matching their lavatory wash-basin. In the 1870s and 1880s, wooden panelling had been used to achieve an *en suite* effect, but from about 1890, exposed ceramic appliances could be matched by their own ornament in relief or under the glaze.

From the 1870s the pace of change in water-closet design had proceeded at an extraordinary rate, and in the mid-1890s no one saw any reason why it should slacken. After all, a new type of water closet – the syphonic closet – had appeared and was generating a lot of interest. Some of the leading makers – Twyford, Shanks and Jennings – had recently launched their own versions and Hatton for one, the Twyford historian, forecast that soon the wash-out and wash-down would make way for this latest innovation for 'all good work'.[57] While in all previous closets, the waste was removed by the sheer force of the flush water, in the syphonic closet it was removed by suction. The first patent for one was taken out by John Gray as early

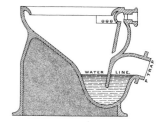

Section of a one-piece 'Deluge' of 1889 with a P or shoot-out trap. It had a water seal of 2 in and was made with Twyford's 'Patent After Flush Chamber'. (*Twyford Bathrooms*)

as 1855. He directed some of the flush water straight to a water-sealed trap below the basin to start a syphonic action which then pulled the waste from the basin.[58] In 1870 an American, John Randall Mann, took out a British patent for a syphon closet with two traps separated by a descending pipe. Further patents followed in Britain throughout the 1870s and 1880s, but most of the development took place in America. In 1876 William Smith of San Francisco introduced a syphon closet activated by a jet of water, and this was then developed by George E. Waring, a prominent American sanitary engineer, who, by 1885 had introduced the 'Decco' syphonic closet.[59] In Britain, however, syphonic closets made virtually no impact until 1894 when, in quick succession, Shanks, Twyford and George Jennings took out patents for their first models.

John Shanks was first with his 'Barrhead' jet-syphon closet patented in March. The jet of water was directed centrally down the trap from the back of the basin.[60] Twyford's design, the 'Twycliffe', was patented in July,[61] and George Jennings's closet just a week later.[62] Twyford employed two jets of water to charge the syphon: one at the base of the pan and the other behind the trap. Both Shanks's and Twyford's versions worked with a single trap – another American innovation[63] – but George Jennings's 'Closet of the Century' retained the double-trap arrangement with a pipe in between from which the air was vented by a so-called 'puff pipe'.

The sudden appearance of these three syphonic closets by leading British makers did not represent any new thinking in closet design – the technology had been in place for some time – but was rather part of a commercial struggle by rival firms to capture the upper end of the market. The syphonic closet was expensive, and with the wash-down closet rapidly consolidating its place mainly as a lower- and middle-priced

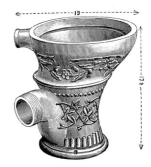

The 'Triple Alliance' wash-down closet. Patented by Freeman Brothers, Battersea, London in December 1892, this closet was designed so that the outlet and inlet could be arranged at different angles to each other. The closet also appears in the 1895 catalogue of Sharpe Brothers, Swadlincote and was probably made by them for Freeman Brothers. (*Sharpe Bros and Co. Ltd, Swadlincote*)

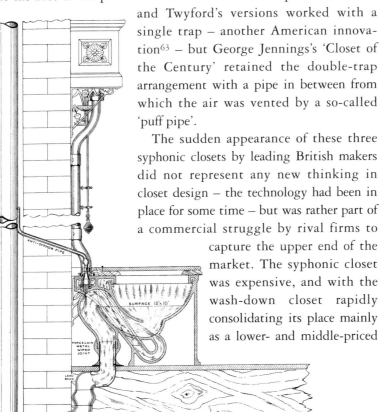

A cross-section of Twyford's single-trap syphonic closet from the 1894 catalogue showing how a jet of flush water entered the base of the bowl to start the syphon.

device, the way was open for a top-quality, all-ceramic pedestal closet to replace the venerable valve closet. The syphonic closet offered several practical advantages over other types. It was practically silent in operation and as the discharge of the foul water from the basin was not dependent upon the force of the flush, their basins were given a larger surface area of water and a deeper seal, which effectively drowned solids and thus deodorised them. Twyford's emphasised this in the publicity for the 'Twycliffe' when it made its debut in their 1894 catalogue: the depth of water in the basin, they claimed, was 7 in and its surface area, 120 sq in. Its water seal was 3½ in and this formed an effective barrier to the passage of sewer gas. The 'Twycliffe' was available in 1894 in Twyford's two most expensive styles of decoration – the 'Venetian' pattern and the classically inspired 'Corinthian' which used coloured slips (liquid clays) to create raised coloured ornament, a technique called 'Pate Dure'. George Jennings's 'Closet of the Century' was rather more traditional in appearance. The flush was operated by a pull-up handle recessed in the wide wooden seat which effectively hid the ugly pipe work at the back. The closet is shown in Jennings's catalogues from about 1900 surrounded by mahogany panelling, which probably appealed to customers with conservative tastes.

The important part played by American sanitary engineers in the development of the syphonic water closet marked the beginning of a new era in sanitaryware manufacture in the United States. In 1886, Glenn Brown, an American architect, wrote, 'Water closets are generally a copy or at least of the same class as closets in the old country. The Bramah, the Jennings, the Brighton and hopper closets have their counterparts in this country, varying only in slight and unimportant details.'[64] Companies such as Jennings, Doulton and Twyford exported sanitaryware to America and maintained agencies in New York. The 1888 catalogue of the J.L. Mott Ironworks, New York, included the English 'Dolphin' wash-out closet – 'an ornament to any bathroom' – and the 'Inodoro', another wash-out model that they described as 'a beautiful piece of porcelain made for us in England'.[65] But in the 1880s some of those British workers, affected by an economic recession, emigrated to the USA and assisted in the development of ceramic sanitaryware manufacture in New Jersey and at a new town, Pottersville, Wisconsin. By the turn of the century, water-closet innovations were occurring on almost a daily basis. The US Patent Office received 350 applications for new water-closet designs between 1900 and 1932. Two of the first granted in the new century were to two New Englanders, Charles Neff and Robert Frame who, it is claimed in America, were the first to produce a syphonic wash-down or reverse-trap closet that was

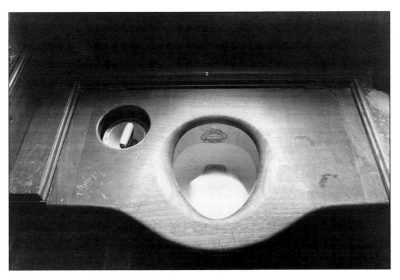

The 'Closet of the Century', a syphonic closet introduced by George Jennings in 1894, installed in East Cliff Hall, Bournemouth, built between 1898 and 1901 for Merton Russell-Cotes, a local hotel proprietor and art connoisseur. The house subsequently became the town's museum and art gallery. (*Russell-Cotes Art Gallery and Museum*)

widely adopted in the United States.[66] This was a single-trap syphonic closet which relied on narrowing the bore of the trap to create a vortex in the water which then started the syphonic action.

In Britain, the choice of water closets was probably never greater than in the 1890s. The old pan closet was generally discredited but remained in production. Hopper closets, whether long or short, were also known to be insanitary, but they were still on sale in 1910. The wash-out closet was also past the peak of its popularity, but Twyford still had the 'Unitas' in their catalogue of 1910, although by then it was reduced to a plain white pedestal in accordance with early twentieth-century sanitary principles. In Britain, wash-out closets remained in use in hospitals because of the ease of examining the faeces in the shallow pan. They continued to be made for the export market – principally to the Low Countries and Germany where they remained popular for the same reason. For 'high-class work', there was a choice between the newly introduced syphonic closet and the traditional valve closet that retained a small but faithful following. Various improvements were made to valve closets in the late nineteenth century, but the device was still recognisably Bramah's design of 1778. Hellyer's 'Optimus' was still on sale in the early 1930s, and one of the last makers was Thomas Crapper and Co. who made them until about 1939. A few continue in use at the time of writing: Twyford Bathrooms continue to service some at the royal palaces. Syphonic closets were widely adopted in the USA, but never completely replaced the wash-down as Hatton had predicted. They were not without their own particular problems: the jet orifice in the bowl of the 'Twycliffe', for example, could become clogged with dirt

Toilet paper

THE ROMANS used sponges, Henry VIII used a flannel 'to wipe his nether end' while in the eighteenth century, the Earl of Chesterfield advised his son to use pages from books of poetry. Ordinary people used bunches of hay, cotton waste or old newspapers torn into squares that were strung together or impaled on a spike.

Specially made toilet paper first appeared in the second half of the nineteenth century: Gayety's Medicated Paper Co. started business in America in 1857. The first British patent for toilet paper was taken out by F. Feichtinger in 1863 and specified the use of unsized paper treated with a mixture of boiled willow bark, 'china bark' and gall nuts. Further patents followed in the late 1880s and 1890s and most specified the addition of various substances to the pulp including carbolic acid, eucalyptus and pine oils, galls and opium to render the paper antiseptic and to give it disinfectant properties.

The Scott Paper Co. of Philadelphia is credited with inventing rolled toilet tissue in 1879, and in the following year the British Perforated Paper Co. was formed by W.J. Alcock to make Bronco. By the early 1880s toilet paper was being made with perforations at set distances, but in June 1884 *The Ironmonger* reported that the Sanitary Paper Co. had introduced rolls of toilet paper prepared in lengths of 500 feet without perforations. Instead, the required length of paper was torn from the roll using a cutter along the front edge of a specially made bronzed holder. Textured and wrinkled or crepe-like toilet papers were the subject of patents in the late 1880s and 1890s and paper printed with advertisements had appeared by 1899.

Hard toilet papers such as Bronco and Izal dominated the market until the 1950s but then gave way to soft absorbent tissues. Now the most successful brand is Andrex, originally introduced as a man's handkerchief in 1936. In 1942 it was launched as a toilet tissue by the Scott Paper Co. and named after St Andrew's Mill in Walthamstow where it was first made. Sales of Andrex were apparently boosted by Hollywood movie stars who refused to use hard toilet

paper (known as shinies) and insisted that their studios were supplied with Andrex for their visits. Andrex was produced in colour for the first time in 1957 and in 1961 was established as the leading brand in the UK. In 1971 Andrex became the first toilet tissue to gain permission to advertise on television and the celebrated Andrex puppy commercial made its first television appearance the following year.

In 2002 the toilet tissue market was worth £766 million – five times greater than the combined shampoo and conditioner market and four times that for toothpaste. As virtually no one would now think of wiping themselves with squares of old newspapers, hay – or even pages from books of poetry – the market for toilet tissue is unusual in that market penetration is nearly 100 per cent. With a value share of around 27 per cent, Andrex, now produced by Kimberley-Clark (an American company founded in Wisconsin in 1872), remains the most popular brand in the UK.

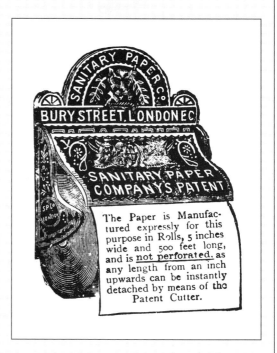

and the reduced bores of the wash-down syphonic were liable to blockages if misused.

It was the simpler and cheaper wash-down which was adopted almost universally in early twentieth-century Britain. The 'fin de

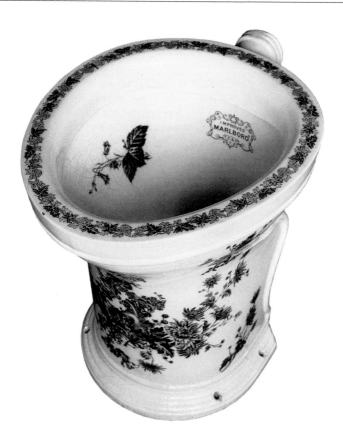

The 'Improved Marlboro'
pedestal wash-down closet by
Thomas Crapper and Co.,
c. 1895.

siecle' designs in colour and relief ornament began to give way after 1900 to closets made chiefly of white earthenware or white enamelled fireclay, usually with a cutaway front in place of the full-front pedestal. Variety of form was further reduced by the publication of guidelines by the British Standards Institution: these provided recommended dimensions for the exterior and the interior of the basin and trap – in the interests of sanitary hygiene, not aesthetics.[67] No single sanitary engineer can take the credit for the 'invention' of the wash-down; rather, through the muddle of innovations and fashions of the 1870s and 1880s, it slowly emerged from its humble origins as a variant of the hopper closet. It is fitting that in the egalitarian twentieth century, the most widely used water closet had started life as a 'back stairs' device used by 'mechanics and domestics'.

CHAPTER EIGHT

Flushes of Water

cisterns and tipplers

Water closets could function – as all early types had to – without a system of mains sewers, but they could not work without a plentiful supply of water to flush out the pan. The flush water had to contend with many different kinds of waste. In 1878, according to Dr Chesshire from Birmingham – an opponent of the water closet system – this could include 'all the faecal matter, viscid and tenacious as that substance is, all the paper, hair, dish cloths and other solid matters'.[1] These other solid matters could consist of just about anything. In mid-Victorian London Henry Mayhew described how sewer hunters made a living by collecting all sorts of solid matter – including valuables such as coins, silver plate and items of jewellery washed down from house drains; some of which had probably been inadvertently dropped into the closet.[2] Apples, sponges, cotton waste, grease or plumber's 'smudge' were placed in closets by manufacturers to test the efficiency of new models. One particularly exacting test, employed by Thomas Crapper and Co., used so-called 'air vessels' – pieces of paper, twisted and folded into the shape of Christmas crackers – which floated on the water and as a result were particularly difficult to flush away.[3] With the exception of syphonic closets, where the foul water in the basin was sucked out, the effectiveness of the flush depended upon the force and volume of the flush and how it was distributed inside the basin. The greater the supply of water, the greater the efficiency of the closet – but for much of the nineteenth century, domestic water supplies were insufficient in many parts of Britain to provide flush water for closets. In the second half of the century, piped water supplies reached many urban homes, but this was not the solution that might have been expected: the water companies were opposed to what they saw as the profligate waste of water pouring through water closets. There was, therefore, a basic tension between the sanitaryware manu-facturers, whose appliances worked best with plentiful water

'The great object to be secured in the delivery of water to the closet is that it shall completely wash and flush out the basin and traps.'
J. Bailey Denton, 1877.

supplies, and the water companies who strove to curb consumption. From the 1870s the water companies exerted considerable influence on the design of cisterns, and the drive to reduce water wasting was to lead to a new type of water closet – the tipper closet.

Before the 1850s houses with a constant supply of piped water formed an exclusive minority. In many towns and villages water had to be collected from public wells – picturesque, perhaps, but hardly convenient. In Liverpool in the 1840s houses in the poorer districts had to rely on communal stopcocks in courtyards or the street; the water was only turned on for a quarter of an hour every other day at either six in the morning or eleven at night.[4] In Birmingham in the early 1870s water was so scarce, according to the city's mayor, Joseph Chamberlain, that the poor were reduced to stealing it from others or drawing it from contaminated wells. The indifferent quality of well

'One tap with a cock serves to supply the whole thirteen houses.' Hector Gavin on Martha Court, Bethnal Green, 1848.

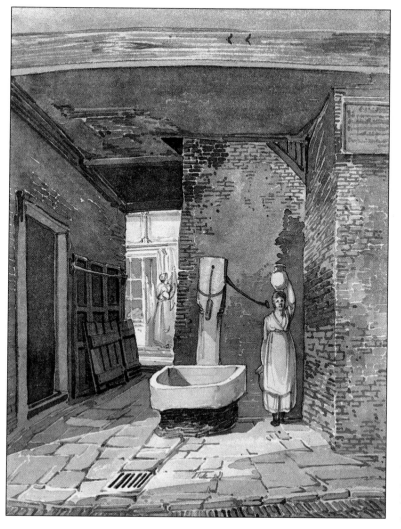

Scenes like this were common across Britain in the early nineteenth century as householders had to resort to public pumps to obtain their water. Women and servants could be seen carrying the water to their homes in pails or in pitchers balanced on their heads, as seen here in this watercolour by Hugh O'Neill of the Pithay in the centre of Bristol in 1821. (*Bristol City Museum and Art Gallery*)

water – and occasionally company water, where it was on hand –
represented a major danger to health. Of course, it was the volume of
water available – and not its purity – which was critical to the use of
water closets and in many parts of the country, erratic and inadequate
supplies represented a major obstacle to their adoption. Thus dry
privies and middens remained common in many towns, and in the

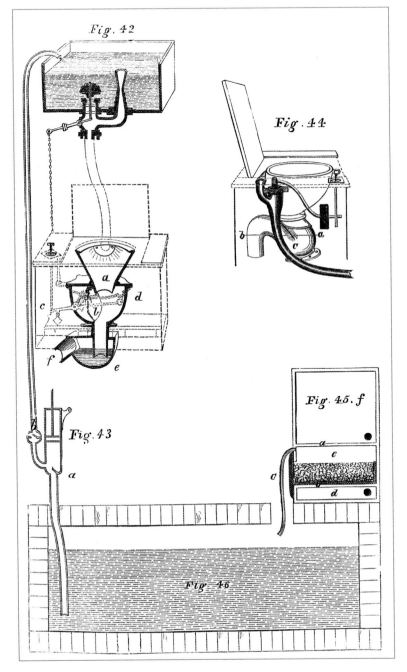

A diagram from Walsh's
Manual of Domestic Economy,
1857, showing a pan closet
connected to an overhead
cistern supplied from an
underground tank containing
rain water. The water enters
the tank after first passing
through a filter (fig. 45) and is
then pumped up to the
overhead tank by the force
pump (fig. 43). The diagram
shows the apparatus in action:
the pull-up action of the
handle has tipped the pan of
the closet down into the
receiver which leads to the
D trap. Simultaneously, the
weighted valve in the water
tank has lifted due to the
pulling of the chain connected
to the handle and flush water is
rushing down the pipe,
entering the basin behind the
spreader.

countryside the shortage of water was undoubtedly a major factor in the success of the earth closet after 1860.

Rain was another source of water. The poor collected it in water butts, while in some larger houses, it was conducted through internal lead-lined conduits to storage tanks in the cellars. The water was usually then pumped up to a cistern connected to the water closets every day by a servant. Lord Chesterfield had such a self-contained water supply in his London house at 45 Grosvenor Square in the early 1730s: there was a force pump in the garden which conveyed water up to a cistern above a water closet on the first floor.[5] The sale particulars of Walcot House in Bath in September 1833 included 'a very large tank of soft water with force pump' in the basement that supplied two water closets.[6] The rain water was suitable for flushing water closets, but was not usually considered fit for human consumption – and in larger eighteenth-century houses deep wells provided purer water suitable for drinking and the preparation of food. Advertisements for good-quality houses to let in newspapers of the late eighteenth century occasionally refer to houses with 'both kinds of water': well water for drinking and rain water for scullery use, laundering and flushing the water closet.

Between the 1840s and the 1860s, the availability of piped water improved markedly in many towns as new sources of water were secured. Some were at a considerable distance from the towns they served; the water was conducted through miles of cast-iron pipes using gravity, and if the water had to be pumped uphill steam power was employed. Some of the suppliers were privately owned, such as the Bristol Water Works Co., formed in 1846: they were encouraged by the rise in the demand for water which, in this period, could largely be attributed to the increasing popularity of the water closet among the better-off. But many waterworks were municipally run, and between the 1830s and 1870, the number of waterworks under municipal control increased from just eleven to sixty-nine. For local authorities the impetus to improve water supplies came from the need to raise local standards of public health in the light of the often unflattering findings contained in sanitary reports of the mid-nineteenth century. The rapid increase in the populations of many large towns at this time only further aggravated an already dire situation. In 1842 Edwin Chadwick had been clear that without water there could be no improvement in sanitary conditions. Improving standards of cleanliness within the town was also a matter of civic pride, and the construction of a handsome Italianate or Gothic pumping station filled with gleaming architectural ironwork, steam engines and pumps formed the visible expression of the local commitment to improving public health.

In Liverpool, local-authority control of the water supply was established in 1847, and by 1857 the city was being supplied with water from Rivington Pike on the edge of the Pennines, between Blackburn and Burnley.[7] In Glasgow, the water supply came under municipal control in 1855, and waterworks at Loch Katrine, 34 miles from the city, were opened by Queen Victoria in October 1859. By March the following year the supply was general throughout the city.[8] Queen Victoria also opened a new reservoir serving Aberdeen in 1866. The city's population increased by 19 per cent between 1861 and 1871, but the consumption of water in this period doubled. Much of this was due to the increasing use of water closets: in 1861 the city acquired the powers by act of Parliament to compel householders to fit a sink and water closet where the water supply in the street was within 10 yd of the house. The result was the virtual eradication of dry privies.[9] There were similar results elsewhere: the laying of water stimulated demand and encouraged the adoption of water closets and, from the 1870s, fitted bathrooms.

There were fixed charges for the use of water according to the size of the house. For example, on a house with a yearly rent of £20 the Bristol Water Co.'s annual rate was £1, on a house of £50 rental it was £2 and on a £100 house it was £3. In common with other companies, the Bristol Water Co. made an extra charge for baths and water closets.[10] But many encountered difficulties in maintaining the supply in the face of a sharp increase in demand. Water supplies were not always constant. In London, where the supply was in the hands of eight private companies, large areas of the metropolis lacked a constant supply in the 1880s,[11] although the companies managed to pay their shareholders an average dividend of 7 per cent.[12] For the municipally run companies, commercial performance was less important. In Birmingham, the energetic mayor, Joseph Chamberlain, who had wrested control of the water company from private hands in 1875, was not interested in making a profit from water – any surplus income was to go in the reduction of the price in the interests of public health.[13] But it was clearly of prime importance to all companies – private and public alike – that water was used carefully.

Waste was the enemy. By the 1840s, through the use of inadequate taps, leaking cisterns and the careless and extravagant use of flush water, waste had emerged as a major problem for many companies. An act of Parliament in 1847 introduced fines for wastage. It laid down that 'every person supplied with water . . . who shall suffer any cistern, pipe, ball or stop cock to be out of repair, so that the water supply shall be wasted, shall forfeit . . . a sum not exceeding five pounds'.[14] In 1871 the Metropolis Water Act

'A constant supply of water would only form an inducement to waste.'
William Eassie, 1872.

introduced further restrictions to prevent the waste of water. In Glasgow, finding that a 'considerable quantity' of the new water supply was running to waste, the water commissioners created a body of some twenty inspectors to examine fittings.[15] Later in the century some companies were compelled to augment their existing sources to meet the increased demand. In 1880 Liverpool authorised a scheme to bring water to the city from the upper River Vyrnwy in Powys. When it was completed in 1892 it was the largest artificial lake in Europe. In 1903 Glasgow increased the depth of waters in Loch Katrine, and in Bristol the company obtained parliamentary approval to build a reservoir at Blagdon in the Mendips which was completed in 1901.

So how did the legislation influence the design of water closets and cisterns? Until the mid-nineteenth century, flushing cisterns consisted of large storage tanks made of slate or wood-lined with sheet lead. They were usually located high up in the house – in an attic or loft space – out of sight of the closet and typically held a day's supply of flush water: perhaps between 20 and 40 gallons. The flush was released by 'remote control' from the water closet by a system of cranks, pulleys and copper wire, similar to that used to operate servants' bells. The wire was attached to a pivoted lever at the top of the tank that was connected to a simple weighted valve, fitted with a washer in the base of the tank. A tug of the pull handle by the user lifted the valve and the closet was flushed out. The duration of the flush depended on the user: a short, impatient tug of the handle and the closet basin would not be thoroughly cleaned. Conversely, a fastidious user could use an excessive quantity of water, rapidly reducing the day's supply in the tank. Water could also be wasted through a faulty valve – either by jamming open or due to a worn washer. As long as the tank was supplied independently from a basement cistern, the waste of water was purely a domestic matter, but when the water was from a company supply the consequences were more serious.

The laying on of piped water rendered rain-water tanks and force pumps redundant; instead, the flushing tank was fitted with a main's supply governed by a ballcock. A brass or copper ball floated on the water and when the level in the tank fell, the arm connected to the ball opened an inlet valve. Spherical floats used to control a valve were known of early in the eighteenth century. The architect, Sir John Vanbrugh, illustrated one in a sketchbook of about 1720.[16] They were used occasionally in the eighteenth century in conjunction with simple plug cocks where, for example, a tank was supplied with water by gravity. Plug cocks or taps – like the simple wooden taps

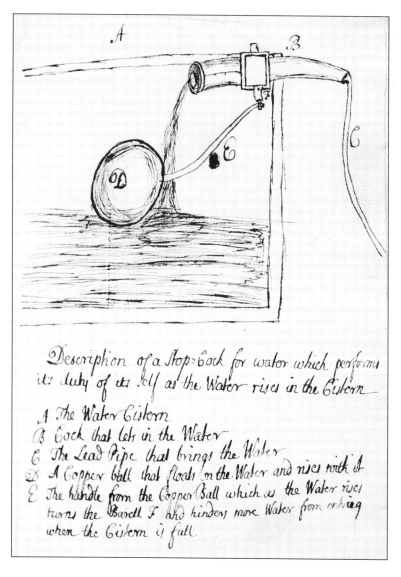

Description of a Stop-Cock for water which performs its duty of its self as the Water rises in the Cistern

A The Water Cistern
B Cock that lets in the Water
C The Lead Pipe that brings the Water
D A Copper ball that floats on the Water and rises with it
E The handle from the Copper Ball which as the Water rises turns the Barrell F and hinders more Water from entring when the Cistern is full

A drawing of a ballcock from Sir John Vanbrugh's 'Designs for Kings Weston House', *c.* 1720. 'Description of a stop-cock for water which performs its duty of itself as the water rises in the cistern [with] a copper ball that floats on the water and rises with it – the handle from the copper ball which as the ball rises turns the barrell and hinders more water from entering when the cistern is full.' (*Bristol Record Office*)

used in barrels – consisted of a cylindrical plug, tapered to fit a conical socket in the body of the cock. The plug had a rectangular opening that was turned in line with the waterway in the socket to allow water to pass through. But they were unsuitable for use with water supplies delivered at constant high pressure. Plug taps closed off the water too suddenly, causing a concussive bursting strain on the pipes, and if the tap was only partially closed, the pressure of water behind it was sometimes sufficient to force it open and cause waste. Moreover, under pressure, they leaked constantly. So, various types of compression – or screw-down – cocks were devised for use with mains water. The Rotherham brass founders, Guest and Chrimes, are credited with first introducing the screw-down cock

and in 1845, Edward Chrimes took out a patent for three designs of high-pressure valves connected to ball floats which could work against the pressure of piped water.[17]

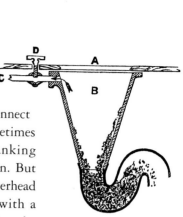

As J.H. Walsh pointed out in 1857, it was even possible 'in towns where water is laid on at high pressure' to do away with the cistern altogether and connect the closet directly to the mains supply. This method was sometimes used with hopper closets which did not have the cranking mechanism needed to operate the valve in an overhead cistern. But lacking the velocity of water discharged suddenly from an overhead cistern, the tap method merely provided the closet basin with a constant supply of water which had little or no effect on scouring the pan. And Walsh conceded that even with the use of various high-pressure valves, such as Jennings's cock with an india-rubber lining, there was a 'great waste' of water.[18]

Diagram of a hopper closet flushed by an ordinary tap (D). The drawing shows the accumulation of waste in the trap and how foul water could be syphoned into the mains pipe (C), and then drawn from the tap in the scullery (E).

The act of 1847 recognised the waste of water caused by continuous leakage from faulty valves and fittings, but not the deliberate waste caused by people propping up the closet handle allowing water to run through for hours on end. From the 1850s hundreds of patents were taken out for valves, cisterns and other devices designed to govern the quantity of flush water admitted to the closet independent of the user. The earliest was patented in 1852 by Frederick Underhay, a sanitary engineer in Farringdon Street, London, and was designed to be attached to valve and pan closets.[19] He called it a 'regulator', and it consisted of a brass or copper cylinder filled with water and containing a piston. The piston was connected to a lever operated from the closet handle that opened the supply valve, thus releasing the flush, when it was lifted. The piston, of course, was raised by the same action, but its descent was delayed by the resistance of the water in the cylinder. So when the closet handle was released the outlet valve of the closet closed instantaneously, but the supply valve remained open until the piston had reached the base of the cylinder. The regulator did not prevent waste, but it ensured that a minimum quantity of water flowed through the closet and – importantly – that an ample supply of water, or 'after-flush', refilled the basin. Underhay also devised regulators which used the resistance of air in a cylinder fitted with a leather diaphragm – these were generally known as 'bellows' regulators.[20] In 1864, he patented a regulator consisting of a slim cylinder with another one inside connected to the supply lever by a spindle that used air pressure to delay the closing of the valve.[21] By the mid-1870s he had devised another similar mechanism which prevented the continuous use of the water supply. This one, again, had a movable cylinder connected

by a spindle to the supply lever and fitted inside a fixed cylinder. A small portion of the flush water was diverted to the device, forcing the inner cylinder upwards until it closed the water-supply valve. The closet could not be flushed again until the water had drained out of a small outlet in the base of the outer casing allowing the inner cylinder to return to its original position.[22]

Underhay's regulators were a success. Pan closets of his design, fitted with the regulator, were installed at the Great International Exhibition held in London in 1862 and, according to the exhibition catalogue, were also in use at the Houses of Parliament, Windsor Castle and the Grosvenor Hotel, Pimlico.[23] They were also widely adopted by other makers. The London brass founders, John Warner

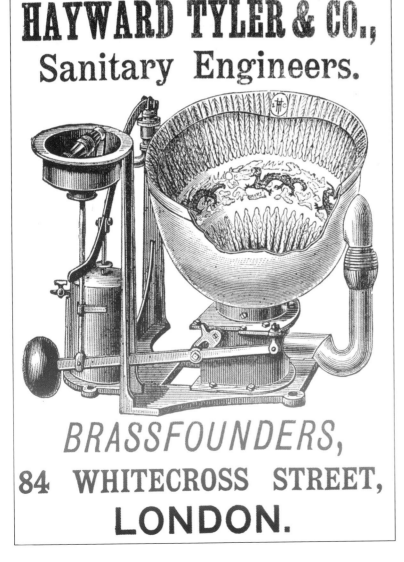

HAYWARD TYLER & CO.,
Sanitary Engineers.

BRASSFOUNDERS,
84 WHITECROSS STREET,
LONDON.

'Every water closet cistern . . . hereafter fitted or fixed in which water supplied by the company is to be used shall have an efficient waste preventing apparatus, so constructed as not to be capable of discharging more than two gallons of water at each flush.' The Metropolis Water Act, 1871, clause 21.

Valve closets made from the 1850s were usually fitted with a regulator or water-waste-preventing valve. This closet, made by Hayward Tyler and Co. is fitted with a regulator connected to the inclined lever controlling the supply valve, which can be seen at the back. The basin has a flushing rim and an overflow connected to the valve box below. The makers are obviously proud of the Japanese-style decoration of the pan. *The Ironmonger,* 26 July 1884. (*Rural History Centre*)

and Sons, for example, featured them in
their 1856 catalogue – not only fitted to
valve and pan closets, but also to cottage
basins and traps flushed directly from the
mains supply. Their 1856 catalogue shows
Underhay's 'Patent Regulator' connected by
a lever to a high-pressure supply valve and
fixed to an enamelled iron basin and trap.[24]
But they were cumbersome devices and
other sanitary engineers turned to the
development of sophisticated regulating
valves that incorporated a 'timing device' to
govern the duration of the flush. In 1856,
Robert Howard patented a regulating valve
that used the resistance of a small quantity
of water diverted from the flush to retard
the movement of a piston attached to the
valve.[25] Similar devices were patented by

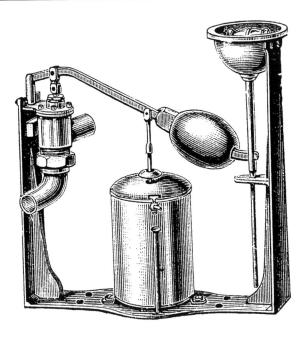

George Jennings in 1858 and J. Tylor and Sons, another London firm
that made something of a speciality of these valves from 1859.[26] The
valves subsequently developed by Tylor included 'waste not' devices
which ensured that the water supply was automatically closed after a
set quantity of water, usually about 2 gallons, had passed through
the closet.[27]

Many of these devices could be used without a cistern and
attached straight to the mains supply. In 1856, Warner and Co.
argued that 'it is necessary for economy that closets should be
attached direct to the main in all . . . cases'.[28] But this was contrary
to the views of the water companies and local boards of health that
were opposed to closets being connected to mains pipes in case foul
water from the closet was syphoned back into the supply. The
Metropolis Water Act of 1871 required that water closets should be
'served only through a cistern or service box . . . and there shall be no
direct communication from the pipes of the company to any boiler,
urinal or water closet'. The act also decreed that 'every water closet,
cistern or water closet service box hereafter fitted or fixed in which
water supplied by the company is to be used shall have an efficient
waste preventing apparatus, so constructed as not to be capable of
discharging more than two gallons of water at each flush'. By the
early 1880s, many local sanitary authorities had passed by-laws based
on this legislation. The law clearly favoured the water-waste-
preventing flushing cistern. Sanitary engineers such as Hellyer
continued to support the use of regulators with valve closets where
water companies permitted their use. But the rapid adoption of the

Regulators were also adapted
for use with simple
earthenware basin and trap
closets. A cast-iron frame
supported the mechanism. The
closet handle, set in its sunken
brass cup, is seen on the right.
This is connected to the
weighted lever that operates
the supply valve on the left.
The spindle of the cylindrical
regulator in the centre is
connected to the lever and
slows its descent to the closed
position, thus regulating the
amount of flush water.

all-ceramic water closet from the late 1870s also encouraged the use of overhead cisterns: pedestal closets had no valves and, therefore, no cranking mechanism to which a regulator could be attached. The mechanics governing the flush moved up to the overhead cistern.

The cistern was no longer placed out of sight in the roof, but usually supported on brackets about 5 or 6 ft above the basin and, in effect, became an integral part of the appliance. The use of small cisterns within reach of the user also changed the way the flush was operated. Instead of pulling up a handle recessed in the seat, the flush was now operated by pulling down on a handle suspended from a chain that was connected directly to a lever operating the flush mechanism in the tank. 'Pulling the chain' was about to enter the English language as an essential item of sanitary parlance. The earliest handles were simple loops of iron or brass, but it was not long before handsome ceramic handles often inscribed 'pull once' became popular.

Waste-preventing cisterns first appeared in the mid-1850s. The simplest measure was to add a smaller cistern fed from the main tank which could hold just enough water for a single flush. But if the main tank was supplied with constant pressurised water, it was still possible for waste to occur through misuse of the flush, or through a faulty valve in the smaller cistern. An arrangement was required, therefore, which would ensure that the mains supply was closed during the flushing of the appliance. A simple solution, described by J.H. Walsh in 1857, consisted of a vertical arm attached to the weighted valve in the cistern. When the valve was raised by a pull of the handle, it held the ballcock up preventing fresh water entering the cistern until it had closed. According to Walsh, this cistern was made by the well-known London sanitary engineer, George Jennings: it held between 1 and 1½ gallons and could be purchased for 35*s*.[29] Walsh called it a 'Water Waste Preventer', a term often abbreviated to 'WWP', which was to become universal in the world of Victorian sanitary engineering.

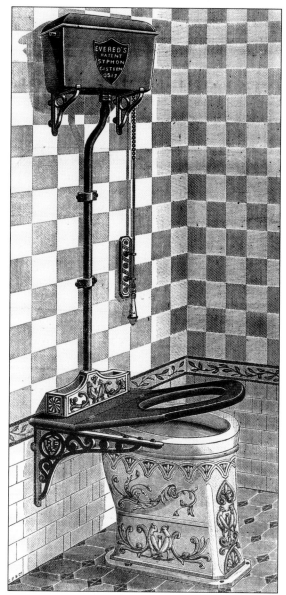

The adoption of the pedestal closet went hand in hand with that of the 2-gallon water-waste preventer activated by a chain and pull. Here we see the 'Sussex' wash-down closet with lift-up seat and ceramic paper box by Evered and Co., London and Birmingham, connected to their patent syphon cistern. *The Ironmonger*, 17 September 1892. (*Rural History Centre*)

The simple method of preventing waste by holding the ballcock up and thus closing the mains supply valve was adapted by other makers besides Jennings. The 'Single Chambered Water Waste Preventer Cistern' of Messrs Stone, for example, worked this way,[30] but there was still a risk of waste if the valve leaked in its seating. So sanitary engineers devised more complicated cisterns that could only release a predetermined quantity of water – and not a drop more. One solution, widely adopted from the 1850s, involved dividing the cistern into two unequal compartments: the larger one formed a reserve and contained the mains supply and a ballcock. The smaller chamber contained the water required for one flush and was fitted with an outlet to the closet pan. A second outlet connected the two compartments and both were controlled by a weighted valve. The valves were operated by a lever pivoted across the central partition so that it was impossible for them to be open at the same time. So when the flush water was released, the outlet between the two chambers remained closed and the water level in the reserve chamber remained constant. When the outlet valve to the closet closed, then the other valve opened. The flushing chamber was then replenished from the reserve ready for the next action of the closet and as the water dropped in the reserve chamber, the ballcock opened to allow fresh mains water to enter. In the mid-1870s, J. Tylor and Sons made a cistern divided into three compartments that they called their 'After Flush Waste Preventing Closet Cistern': a small third chamber was added to provide an after-flush to ensure that the closet was trapped by a water seal.[31]

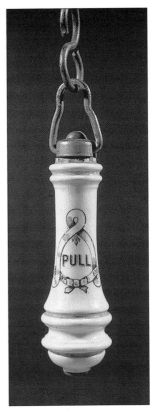

Ceramic pull handle with a transfer-printed design registered in 1887.

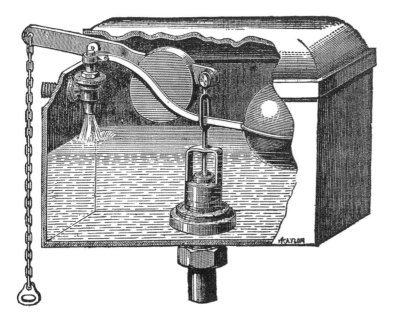

Stone's 'Single Chambered Water Waste Preventer Cistern' of *c.* 1876. The cut away drawing shows how the weighted valve at the bottom of the cistern was connected to the arm of the ballcock so that when the valve lifted to release the flush the arm of the float was held up, preventing mains water entering until the valve dropped.

Single or multiple-compartment cisterns effectively set a limit on the amount of water used for each flush. But they were complicated. There were many moving parts that could go wrong, and as the outlet valve would close when the chain was released, it was still possible for a careless user to terminate the flush prematurely. So cisterns were developed which operated on a 'pull and let go' principle to ensure that regardless of the duration of the pull on the chain, a set amount of flush water would be released by using syphonic action. The syphon in a cistern usually consisted of a pipe bent over above the water level in the cistern. The long leg of the syphon extended through the base of the cistern to form the flush pipe to the closet while the mouth of the shorter leg lay near the bottom of the water in the tank. If some of the water in the cistern was forced up over the bend or elbow at the top of the long arm, a partial vacuum was created that would start the syphonic action. The water in the cistern was then drawn down the pipe to the closet basin until the level dropped below the end of the short leg of the syphon pipe. Thus almost any pull on the chain was enough to start the syphonic action: there was no longer the risk of the closet receiving less than a full quantity of flush water. Equally, holding onto the chain after the flush had been discharged made no difference either, as the cistern could not be used again until it had refilled.

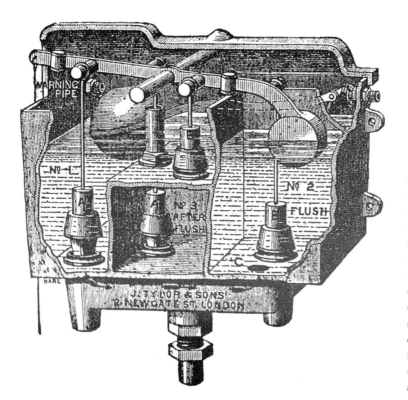

The 'After Flush Waste Preventing Cistern' of J. Tylor and Sons, *c.* 1876, an ingenious device with three compartments and two pairs of valves that opened alternately. The reserve chamber is on the left, the flushing chamber on the right and a small after-flush chamber in the centre. When the lever was pulled to activate the cistern, the valve in the flushing chamber lifted releasing the water, while the valve at the top of the after-flush chamber also opened, allowing water in from the reserve chamber. When the lever was released, these valves closed and the other two opened, one supplying the after-flush to the closet and the other allowing water to pass from the reserve chamber to the flushing chamber by a pipe at the bottom.

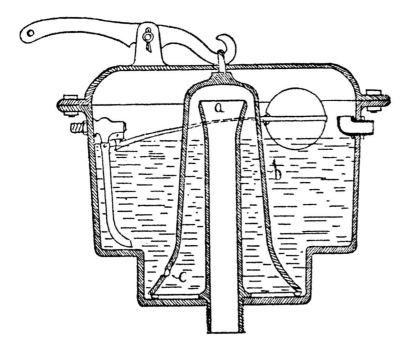

A section of a valveless bell-syphon cistern showing the characteristic bottom well containing the bell. When the bell was raised by pulling the lever and released, it returned to the position shown in the diagram, forcing most of the water in the well over the top of the standpipe. This started the syphonic action. The diagram shows one method of subduing the noise associated with these cisterns: a hole is drilled near the base of the bell (at c) to allow air in gradually before syphonage ceased.

From the 1850s sanitary engineers devised many ways of charging the syphon. The earliest patent for a syphonic cistern was taken out by George Jennings in 1854; it contained a weight on the end of a lever which was depressed to raise the water level above the bend of the syphon.[32] Some cisterns used a valve that lifted the water down the open flush pipe to start the syphonic action. But valves of any sort in a cistern were a source of weakness: over time, the rubber or leather washer fitted to the valve would wear and cease to form a watertight seal; grit or lime deposits could also impair the efficiency of a valve. Jennings's syphonic cistern of 1854 had no valves and was an effective water waste preventer, and yet between 1855 and 1866 only three patents were taken out for syphon discharge cisterns while fifty were taken out for improvements to valve-operated models. It was not until the late 1870s that patents for syphonic cisterns began to outnumber those for cisterns that used valves.

The 1870s saw the development of valveless syphonic water-waste preventers that won the approval of water companies and local boards of health throughout the country. The simplest and most popular type was the bell cistern which had appeared by 1874.[33] It contained a bell or dome with a flared edge placed over the upright leg of the syphon and connected to the lever and chain. The syphonic action was started by pulling and releasing the chain which lifted and then dropped the bell forcing water over the top of the down pipe. The bell was placed in a circular well in the bottom of the cistern. It was important that the sides were close to the bell, so that as it fell water was forced up and over the pipe or leg. The well also had the advantage that when syphonage ceased only a small quantity of water was left in the bottom of the well rather than over the entire base of the cistern, thus maximising the quantity of water discharged.

Syphonic cisterns that were charged by the action of a loose-fitting piston or movable disc in a cylinder were also developed in the 1870s. The cylinder was connected to the end of the short leg of the syphon, so that when the lever was pulled, the piston either lifted or forced water from the cylinder over the syphon bend. The valveless syphonic cistern was effective and economical. Once the syphon was charged, exactly the same quantity of water – usually 2 gallons – was delivered every time, regardless of whether the handle was held down or released. Waste, therefore, was impossible.[34]

The limit of 2 gallons of water set by many water companies from the 1870s almost certainly influenced water-closet development. For some types of closets, 2 gallons was hardly sufficient to ensure a thorough cleaning. The limitations of the pan closet, for example, became more apparent once the use of the 2-gallon cistern became commonplace. T. Mellard Reade, lecturing on 'How to Drain a House' to the Liverpool Architectural Society, said, 'I consider the pan closet objectionable, especially since the introduction of the two gallon regulating cistern has increased the difficulty of getting the after flush to fill the pan.'[35] The 2-gallon limit may also have exposed the tendency of wash-out closets to harbour dirt. Nevertheless, in 1884, Charles Winn and Co. claimed their 'Acme' cistern was 'suitable for use with the various patterns of patent closet pans now so much in vogue, such as Bostel's "Excelsior", Woodward's "Wash-out" . . . Twyford's "National" and Sharpe's "Patent Pan"'.[36] Wash-down closets were easier to flush out with 2 gallons, and so the water regulations may have further encouraged the more general adoption of this type from the late 1880s. Some sanitary engineers, however, reacted angrily to the restrictions imposed by the water companies. In 1877 S. Stevens Hellyer wrote, 'Two gallons to carry away a deposit in a wc through scores of feet of soil pipe and drainage, flush these out after its passage and cleanse the whole! This is about as difficult as making bricks with straw.'[37] And he continued, 'Every sanitarian should lift up his voice against the limitation of water to such sanitary fixtures and never cease crying, like Oliver Twist, for more water and until a quantity double or even treble the present amount is allowed for wcs.' But there was little point in the sanitarians crying about the problem. They had to follow the regulations.

Cisterns, like water closets, were accorded trade names and some even acquired worldwide fame. Many were named after the towns or

'The Metropolitan cistern . . . is admirably adapted for use with the ordinary or pan basins and traps. . . .'
Beck and Co., 1884.

boroughs where they had been adopted by the water authorities. Beck and Co.'s piston-operated syphonic cistern of the 1880s, for example, was called the 'Metropolitan', a name that recognised – or rather capitalised on – the fact that it had been adopted by the largest water companies in London and the provinces.[38] T. and W. Farmiloe named one of their valveless cisterns the 'Westminster',[39] while Milton Syer called their bell syphon the 'Peckham', after the location of their works.[40] Advertisements of the 1880s for the London makers, Hayward Tyler and Co. and A. Emanuel and Sons of Marylebone Lane, both made much of the fact that their cisterns had been passed by the New River Co., one of the eight private water companies in the capital.[41] In 1889 W.H. Gummer and Co., of Rotherham, advertised the fact their 'Niagara' syphonic cistern had been approved by Manchester Corporation.[42] In 1892 Charles Winn and Co. boasted that over 50,000 of their 'Acme' syphonic cisterns were in use, having sold 7,819 in 1891. One of the most celebrated of all was the 'Levern', a bell syphon cistern made by Shanks: in 1904 the company claimed this was 'the simplest form of valveless syphon cistern that has yet been produced'.[43] The company also pointed out that it complied with the regulations of the most important water companies or boards 'all the world over'. In 1895 Shanks won a large contract from the Metropolitan Board of Works in Melbourne, Australia to provide 8,000 cisterns, and over a period of years supplied so many cisterns to Argentina that there cisterns became known simply as 'Shanks'. Large numbers of cisterns were also exported by Shanks to India, Egypt and Denmark.[44]

Overhead cisterns tended to match the closets they served, which meant they ranged from the plain and purely functional to the glamorous and expensive. The simplest were made of unadorned cast iron or deal, the cheapest of woods, lined with lead. These were the cisterns most likely to be found connected to cheap basins and traps in cane and white fireclay, but for the most expensive closets, a better class of cistern was usually available. For example, in their 1893 catalogue, Shanks illustrated the 'Tubal' closet with raised 'acanthus' ornament connected to their 'Reliable' waste preventer. This valveless bell-syphon cistern held the usual 2 gallons of water and was embellished with a florid Renaissance-style relief design. The cistern was 'nicely japanned' – indian red was popular – with the raised pattern picked out in gold. The 'Reliable' was also made in mahogany with a copper lining.[45] But Twyford's went one better, by matching their top-quality models of the 1890s – the 'Deluge' and the 'Twycliffe' – with cisterns given a 'porcelain' casing. The cistern was provided with the same coloured-relief ornament as the pedestal and the paper box. Cisterns were usually supported by decorative

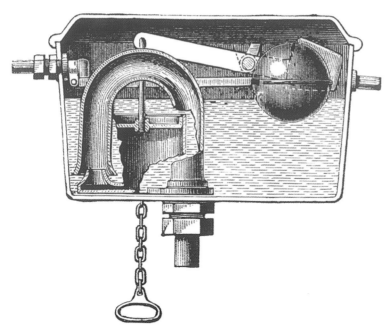

The 'Metropolitan', a piston-type syphon cistern manufactured by Beck and Co., Southwark, London. Patented in 1882, it had no valves and no perishable materials such as rubber or leather. When the chain was pulled a loosely fitted piston in a cylinder forced a jet of water into the syphon pipe, which was then instantly charged and started. Two gallons of water was delivered to the water closet whether the handle was held down or released. *The Ironmonger*, 10 March 1884. (*Rural History Centre*)

cast-iron brackets painted to match the seat brackets, but in about 1890 Thomas Crapper introduced a distinctive water-waste preventer with a shallow, domed lid that was screwed directly to the wall.

Cisterns working on the 'pull and let go' principle made effective water-waste preventers, but the chain had to be pulled first, and not everyone bothered. And if there was one thing worse than the waste of water in closets, it was the use of none at all. From the early days of water closets, self-acting types were devised which could flush independently of the user. William Law's patent of 1796 – the first to feature a pan closet – was actually for a self-acting water closet flushed by rising from the seat.[46] Other self-acting closets relied on foot pedals, and in 1833 J.C. Loudon described a door-action closet where the cable to the cistern was attached to the door.[47] Fully automatic cisterns that flushed periodically, independent of the use of the closet, were also applied to closets and urinals, especially in public and institutional buildings such as schools and hospitals. Many relied on a tipping tank to release the water: these scoop-shaped tanks were balanced on lugs at the side and slowly filled from a dripping tap. Trough closets operated by tipper tanks, known as 'tumbler closets' were in use by the early 1870s in the poor districts of Leeds and Birkenhead. When they were nearly full they overturned, sending their contents down the flush pipe. Cisterns with tipping tanks featured in numerous patents during the second half of the nineteenth century, but the idea was nearly as old as water closets themselves. The closet that John Aubrey saw at the home of

Sir Francis Carew at Bedington, Surrey, in 1673, was flushed by a tipping tank which he likened to a 'bit of a shovel'.[48]

In 1887, a Burnley brick and tile manufacturer, James Duckett, applied the tipping tank to water closets without a cistern and produced a new type of water closet, the tipper closet or 'tippler'. Duckett called them 'Automatic Slop Water Closets' and as the name implied, the tank was filled, not from the mains, but with slop water drained from the kitchen or scullery sink. The tipping tank was made of stoneware and usually held 3 gallons. The position of the tipping tank varied, but it was often located below a grid in the backyard where it could also collect roof and surface water. When the tank was almost full it tipped over, sending a powerful flush of water along a trapped stoneware pipe, laid at a fall beneath the yard, to a second water-sealed trap at the base of the closet pan. In his original patent specification of 1887, Duckett confidently asserted that the tipping tank, 'will be found much superior to the ordinary method of flushing water closets as it is not dependent in any way on the care and cleanliness of the person using the closet'.[49]

This much was true – and no water company could deny that this device was extremely economical in its use of water. But was it

A section of a tipper closet from the 1914 catalogue of James Duckett and Sons, Burnley. The kitchen sink is on the left in the house and the closet across the backyard on the right. The water drains from the sink through the yard grid to the tipper tank which tips when it is almost full. The water then flows through the drainpipe set on a slight incline under the yard to the water-sealed trap that is well below the closet.

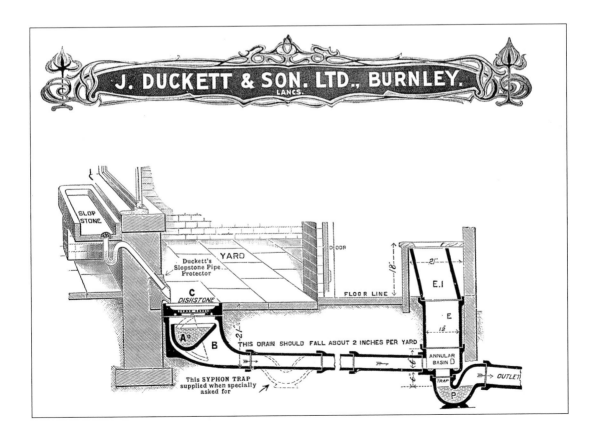

sanitary? Reaction to the closet at the Sanitary Institute's 1887 exhibition at Bolton, where the device was first shown, appears to have been muted. It did not receive an award and reviewing the exhibition, *The Builder* expressed concern that there seemed to be 'no provision for catching grease and solid matters coming from the sink', which over time, could cause a blockage in the trap.[50] The closet pan consisted of an oval stoneware 'pedestal' which was connected at floor level to a vertical 'closet pipe', the other end of which was set into the trap. The distance between the top of the pedestal and the trap was, as the reviewer in *The Builder* noted, two to three times as deep as the ordinary hopper. The trap was obviously not as accessible as those of wash-down closets, which, by 1887 were rapidly gaining ground on other types. Another reservation concerned the cleaning of the interior of the closet. By the 1880s the flushing rim was virtually standard on all ceramic closet pans, but as the water entered a tipper closet level with the trap there was no supply of water to the rim and no provision, therefore, for removing excrement stuck to the sides of the pan. Duckett reacted to the criticisms with a letter to *The Builder*:

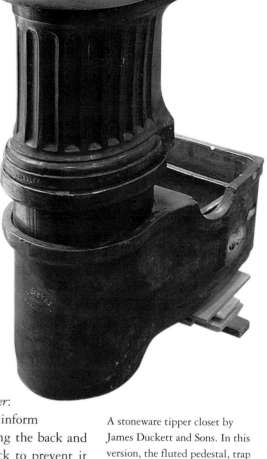

A stoneware tipper closet by James Duckett and Sons. In this version, the fluted pedestal, trap and tipper tank (just visible at the rear) effectively form one unit. Only the pedestal was above ground level. The drainpipe from the house rested on the semi-circular indentation beside the tipper tank, seen on the right. Although they are more particularly associated with Pennine towns, this one came from a house in Chelmsford, Essex.

'with regard to the washing of the pan, we beg to inform you that in practice, we find little if any soil touching the back and sides. The pan extends considerably towards the back to prevent it being soiled.'[51]

Time was to show that this was, in fact, a most insanitary device, but Duckett took out a further twenty-one patents for improvements to his slop-water closets over the next ten years. For example, he reduced the inaccessibility of the trap by bringing the tipper tank indoors and placing it immediately below the sink so that all the pipework leading to the closet and its water-sealed trap were above ground.[52] His model, the 'Rapid', was made this way and was awarded a bronze medal by the Sanitary Institute, at Southampton, in 1899. In a patent of 1892 Duckett constricted the sides of the basin to 'form a quatrefoil passage to arrest salmon tins &c which would otherwise choke up the trap'.[53] Duckett clearly won the support of some local sanitary authorities, water companies and builders, and during the 1890s and the early 1900s, the tipper closet was widely adopted for working-class housing across the border between

Lancashire and Yorkshire. As the tipper closet had to be located below the level of the kitchen sink it was almost invariably found in the backyards of terraced housing; it was never a bathroom fitting. In Pennine towns such as Halifax and Bradford the tipper closet has passed into folklore, notorious for its capacity to give unsuspecting users an unpleasant surprise as 3 gallons of water suddenly crashed into the pan where they quietly sat. One story concerns the author's aunt, Mavis Walton, who as little girl in about 1929, visited family friends in Laisterdyke, Bradford. She retreated quietly to the back-yard closet to avoid having to help with washing the tea things. It was a tipper closet and, of course, it was the washing-up water that caught up with her and gave her quite a shock.[54]

Flushes of water – whether released from a tipper tank or a more conventional overhead cistern – were noisy. The late Victorian water-waste preventer satisfied the water companies and could match the best pedestal closets for splendour, but nothing could hide the noise of one in use. The mechanism of an old and worn cistern might have clanked when the chain was pulled, but this was nothing compared to the mighty crash caused by the water accelerating down the pipe on its way to the pan. A fall of up to 6 feet ensured the water developed sufficient force to thoroughly cleanse the pan and trap, but also announced to everyone present that the closet was engaged. Valveless syphonic cisterns also emitted an annoying gurgling sound – like a child with a straw draining the remnants of a drink from the bottom of a glass – as air mixed with water at the mouth of the syphon pipe. Finally, a shrill penetrating sound was produced as the cistern refilled from the water main. Various modifications were made to cisterns to eradicate these sound effects, including sound-proofing the down pipe and adding a small air pipe which admitted air slowly into the syphon, ending the syphonage gradually without the gurgling.[55]

The most effective solution, however, was to alter the height of the cistern, to place it low, either level with the closet or slightly higher, in which case a short pipe connected the two components. They were called combination closets, and Shanks were early pioneers of the type, including several variations in their 1893 catalogue. Shanks had used a low-level cistern of sorts as early as the 1860s with their 'Number Four' trapless-plunger closet, but in the 1890s, the low-level cistern was invariably combined with a wash-down pan. Shanks claimed in 1893 that 'For wash-down closets this system which we have now very thoroughly proved, is *much superior* to the ordinary system with overhead cistern. The wash-down is coming to be preferred by some sanitarians to the wash-out; and the quick flush

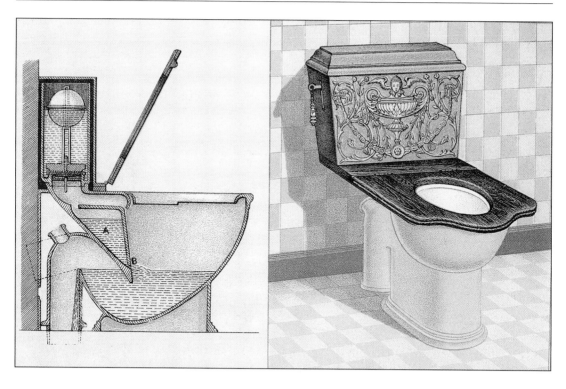

from the above system is a great improvement.'[56] Soon, other makers such as Twyford and Doulton followed with their own combination closets. To counteract the loss of power caused by the low position of the tank, the outlet of the cistern and the inlet of the closet were made larger, and wherever possible, the manufacturers specified the use of a 3-gallon flushing tank. The tanks were originally supplied with short chains and pulls, but Doulton's 'Special Compact Closet' of 1904 had a short lever on the top of the cistern.[57] Low-down tank closets became popular with the Edwardian well-to-do, and after the First World War, the low-level cistern, usually made of ceramicware, became the essential companion of the wash-down closet.

Shanks's 'Combination closet' of 1893 consisting of a close-coupled low-level cistern and wash-down closet in cane and white ware. The front of the cast-iron cistern was heavily decorated with embossed ornament and had a short chain and pull on the side. The diagram on the left shows the after-flush chamber (A) which caught part of the flush and allowed the contents to percolate through the little hole (B) after the flush to ensure the trap was refilled with clean water. (*Mitchell Library, Glasgow*)

CHAPTER NINE

'A Bath in Every Home'

bathrooms in the twentieth century

In 1844 Thomas Hawksley of Nottingham, engineer to the Trent
Water Works, told Edwin Chadwick that he could see a Utopian
future where baths would be 'introduced into the houses of labouring
men for the use of themselves and their families'.[1] In the 1840s the
use of baths was largely restricted to the middle classes, which, it has
been estimated, constituted about 15 per cent of the population in
1850 – and not every middle-class household necessarily owned a
bath. In 1849 Chadwick believed there were entire streets of middle-
class residences without a single bath.[2] After 1850, however, middle-
class bath ownership increased as the middle class itself expanded,
rising to about 20 per cent of the population by 1900.[3] By the early
1880s virtually all new middle-class villas contained a bathroom.[4]
But this still left by far the greater proportion of the population –
perhaps as much as 75 per cent – without a bathroom in 1900. The
adoption of baths by the majority of the population was not
complete until the mid-twentieth century. It was a slow process,
hindered by major obstacles – social, economic and practical –
particularly the scarcity of water, and also by deep prejudices at all
levels of society.

Not everyone, for a start, was as enlightened as Hawksley. In cities
and towns few of the speculative builders responsible for the many
thousands of working-class terraced houses built in the late
nineteenth century and early 1900s thought it worthwhile to
include a bathroom. The quality of housing was governed by the
income it would yield and average working-class rents would not
provide an economic return on the expense of installing a bath and
laying on adequate supplies of hot and cold water. In the countryside
relatively little building of cottage homes took place in the second
half of the nineteenth century. Some enlightened agricultural
landlords, such as the Dukes of Bedford, had built new 'model
cottages 'on their estates from the 1840s and 1850s; but the

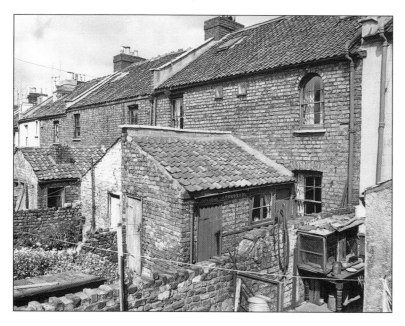

Backyard water closets in Greenbank Avenue, Lower Easton, Bristol, built in about 1898 and photographed in the mid-1950s. The water closets are in the single-storey extensions at the rear of the terrace and have a saw-tooth door that provided ventilation. The window nearest the rest of the house is a back kitchen or scullery, while the door in the gable end provides access to the coal shed. In common with most late Victorian small terraced housing, there was no fitted bath or bathroom. (*Bristol Record Office*)

improvements never went as far as providing a fixed bath: some saw no point and were prepared to say so. As late as 1914 C. Winkworth Allen wrote, 'it is doubtful if a bath should be provided in an agricultural labourer's cottage . . . as a rule there is no demand for baths, and the supply has not hitherto resulted in stimulating one, the bath, when provided, being almost invariably used for storing coal, potatoes, soiled linen etc'.[5] Stories of council-house tenants using the bath to store their coal were legion among 'old ladies in Brighton boarding houses' and others for many years afterwards.[6] In the nineteenth century bathing at home had remained largely the exclusive preserve of the middle classes, and into the twentieth century it is impossible to avoid the conclusion that some wished to keep it that way.

But there may have been a grain of truth in the 'coal in the bath' story. The evidence is fragmentary, but it would appear that in the nineteenth and early twentieth centuries, many ordinary people bathed infrequently, incompletely or not at all. Referring to sponge baths in about 1870, *Cassell's Household Guide* said, 'the majority of people are quite unacquainted with such a thing'.[7] Recalling his childhood in Harpenden in rural Hertfordshire during the 1860s and 1870s, Edwin Grey described how the wooden laundry tub with its sloping sides was used for the children's 'Saturday night bath'. Occasionally it was used by adults too, although, looking back sixty years later, he added, 'a daily or even weekly bath was not then thought to be so essential as it is rightly deemed the case today'.[8] In the early 1870s Emily Kitson, the wife of the Leeds industrialist,

'It is doubtful if a bathroom should be provided in an agricultural labourer's cottage . . . as a rule there is no demand . . . the bath when provided being almost invariably used for storing coal, potatoes, soiled linen etc.'

C. Winkworth Allen, 1914.

James Kitson, found that many young women in the working-class districts of Holbeck and Wortley considered it dangerous to wash their heads; the result was a high incidence of diseases of the scalp among the poor.[9] In the Wigan of the 1930s, George Orwell (1903–1950) found that miners washed the upper halves of their bodies kneeling over a largish basin of water, but did not wash below the waist. Probably a large majority of miners, he wrote, 'are completely black from the waist down for at least six days a week'. He found among the older miners there was even a lingering belief that washing legs could cause lumbago.[10]

Of the practical difficulties which stood in the way of the wider use of baths, shortage of water was probably the greatest. This was especially true of rural areas where piped water supplies were a rarity in the nineteenth and early twentieth centuries. Many cottagers collected rain water from their roofs in water butts: this soft water was ideal for laundry purposes and personal cleaning but supplies depended on the weather – and the size of the roof – and were rarely

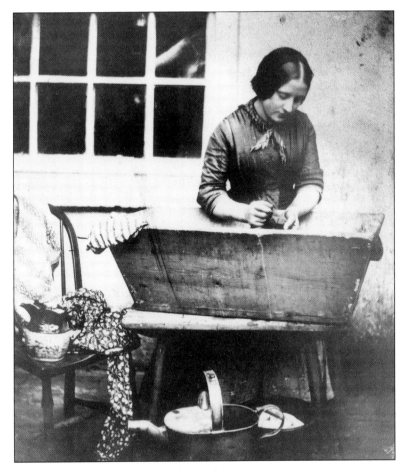

A maid-servant doing the wash in a wooden laundry tub at Redland Villa, Bristol, *c.* 1858. Tubs like this often served as baths in working-class homes – note the hot-water can in the foreground. (*Bristol Record Office*)

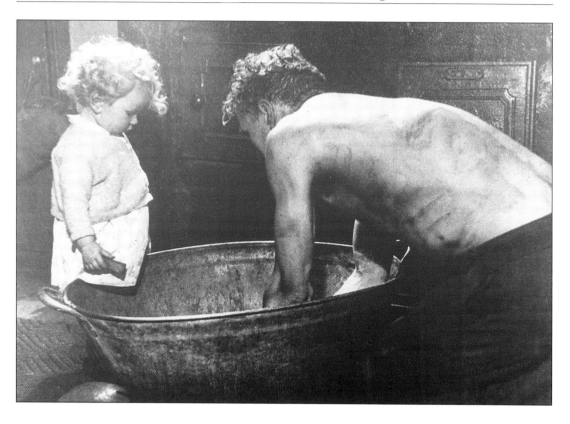

sufficient to meet all the needs of the household. There was usually no alternative but to collect water from a public well or pump. The sheer hard work of operating a pump lever or the windlass of a well and then carrying two full buckets back home – perhaps a distance of 100 yds or more – can hardly have encouraged the use of baths. In towns the supply of mains water reached many working-class homes from the 1860s and 1870s, but supplies were often intermittent and usually confined to a single cold tap on the ground floor. Hot water for preparing baths had to be drawn by hand from the kitchen range.

A shortage of space and the expense of baths were further obstacles to bathing lower down the social scale. Overcrowding typified nineteenth-century working-class housing and large families were crammed into tiny homes. In the countryside two-roomed cottages were common[11] – even the best cottages with three bedrooms usually had no more than a small kitchen and scullery downstairs – and in towns conditions were every bit as cramped in the typical four or six-room terraced house. The bath was rarely taken in bedrooms because of the lack of space between the beds and the trouble of carrying the water upstairs and then down again. Downstairs the congestion could be even worse, leaving little or no room for a bath to be used. These problems persisted into the twentieth century. Of the Wigan

Stripped to the waist and kneeling over a galvanised iron bath, John Davies, a South Wales miner, is watched by his two-year-old daughter, Marion, as he takes his bath in front of the kitchen range at Ferndale in the Rhondda Valley. The arrival of pit-head baths was soon to render scenes such as this a thing of the past.
(*National Museums and Galleries of Wales*)

miners' families in the 1930s, George Orwell wrote, 'it is almost impossible for them to wash all over in their own homes . . . in a tiny living room which contains apart from the kitchen range and a quantity of furniture, a wife, some children and probably a dog there is simply not room to have a proper bath'.[12]

Nevertheless, it would be wrong to assume that because working-class people in the nineteenth century did not bathe that they were filthy and formed the 'great unwashed'. Some practised the simple method of washing all over using buckets and basins by the kitchen fire, in an outhouse or even in the open.[13] In *Lark Rise to Candleford*, Flora Thompson describes how, as a child in the 1880s, she used to wash in the back kitchen or washhouse of their cottage in a north Oxfordshire hamlet. Water from the well was heated over the kitchen range and used sparingly. She also describes the bathing arrangements she encountered a few years later when she lived and worked in the post office of a nearby village. Here a former brewhouse had been converted into a makeshift bathroom: this contained a full-length bath which was used by the neighbouring blacksmiths, who 'on account of the grubby, black nature of their work, needed baths frequently'. They bathed twice a week – on Wednesdays and Saturdays – while Flora bathed on Fridays using a hip bath which was 'stored standing up-ended in a corner when not in use'.[14]

It is likely that habits of cleanliness among the working classes improved towards the later nineteenth century, chiefly due to better education and rising standards of living. Between the 1850s and the 1890s there were significant increases in working-class wages: in 1885, Professor Levi declared in his Report on the Wages and Earnings of the Working Classes that 'working men of the present day are much better off than they were twenty-seven years ago, for all wages are higher'.[15] People had more to spend than they had ever had before, and some of the gains were spent on household goods. Flora Thompson describes how there was a craze for buying washstands and bright, shiny zinc tubs by weekly instalments in the 1880s.[16] Galvanised-iron wash tubs costing just a few shillings became widespread in working-class homes in the late nineteenth and early twentieth centuries. These useful utensils were acquired, it appears, chiefly for laundering clothes, but could also be used for washing the children. In slum properties in the 1930s a zinc bath was often seen hanging up in the backyard on a nail and brought indoors on Saturday evenings when the family would take their turns to have a bath.[17]

Personal hygiene among the poor was improved from the 1870s through increased supplies of tap water and also the greater availability of cheap soap. The removal of the excise duty of 3*d* per pound on soap in 1853 opened the way for manufacturers to introduce more affordable toilet soap. In 1850, 81,796 tons of soap was produced in Britain; by 1881 it is estimated the figure had risen to around 200,000 tons. In the 1880s, William Hesketh Lever (1851–1925), a wholesale grocer, set out to capture the working-class market with cheap, mass-produced soap. His first boil of Sunlight soap was made in Warrington in 1885.[18] The following year he pioneered the sale of bars of soap in individual wrappers; previously soap was cut from a large slab on the shop counter. In 1889, he created new works at Port Sunlight, near Birkenhead on the Mersey and introduced Lifebuoy soap in 1894. He even sought to educate his customers with a pamphlet, 'Sunlight Soap and How to Use it' and the cottages he built for his workers at Port Sunlight were remarkable for the time in containing bathrooms.[19] In larger towns and cities, the presence of multiple retailers brought the price of soap down even further: Boots the chemist had expanded outwards from its Nottingham base in the 1880s, and in 1884 was selling soap in its stores for almost half the price found elsewhere.[20]

From the 1870s, universal education and improved standards of literacy brought working-class families into contact with campaigns to raise standards of personal hygiene. In cities and large towns, middle-class charities provided instruction in domestic economy and

A typical galvanised iron bath tub of the late nineteenth and early twentieth centuries; the importance of bathing children was emphasised in many home manuals of the period. This one was Spark's hammock bath, patented in 1893, for infants, manufactured by Thomas O'Brien and Co., Upper Thames Street, London. *The Ironmonger*, 7 December 1895. (*Rural History Centre*)

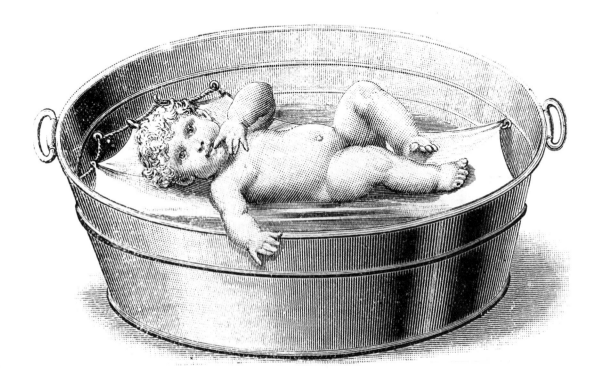

hygiene for the poor. In Leeds, for example, Emily Kitson held classes in sanitation in the Board School in Mann's Field, Holbeck and the Zion School in New Wortley during the winters of 1872 and 1873. Her pupils were young women between the ages of sixteen and thirty who were told that, 'daily ablution is not merely a luxury for "fine folks" but is an essential to comfort and health'.[21] The benefits of keeping clean were also taught to children of school age. A school textbook of 1877, *Domestic Economy: a Class Book for Girls*, emphasised the importance of personal cleanliness: 'The only effective way of cleansing the skin is by the free use of water. A daily bath is an inexpensive luxury, and wherever it can be enjoyed the comfort and health derived from its use will more than repay any amount of trouble or self-denial it occasions.' The book acknowledged the difficulty, 'where there is a proper sense of delicacy and self-respect', of finding space to bathe in crowded houses: 'where the difficulty cannot be overcome, each person can yet thoroughly wash the body every day with a piece of coarse flannel and a little water'.[22] While the book was primarily intended for use in schools it was also considered suitable for those engaged in domestic work. Domestic service was an effective means for the spread of middle-class ways among ordinary people: girls who went into service were inevitably influenced by the way middle-class households were run. Some returned home having absorbed new ideas on furnishings, fashions and domestic economy, including, perhaps, the routine of taking a bath.

For town and city dwellers there was often the alternative of taking a public bath. In 1846 and 1847, two acts of Parliament were passed to encourage the provision of public baths as a valuable means of promoting cleanliness and good health, and from the 1850s municipal baths – which also usually included facilities for laundering and recreational swimming – were provided in many towns and cities. Liverpool had two public baths as early as 1846.[23] By 1915 there were over 343 public baths in Britain maintained by local authorities.[24] Many working people acquired the habit of taking a regular full-length or 'slipper' bath. The public baths located in some of the poorer districts of London such as Shoreditch, Hackney and Bermondsey were well attended. In 1878 the Commissioners of the Baths and Wash Houses in Bermondsey reported that in the twelve months up to March that year, the baths had been used by 101,541 persons including 5,555 women.[25] But not every town was well provided: in 1934 George Orwell found that in the south Yorkshire mining town of Barnsley with a population of 70,000 inhabitants, the public facilities contained just nineteen slipper baths for men.[26]

'Daily ablution is not merely a luxury for fine folks but is an essential to comfort and health.'
Emily Kitson, 1873.

Few working people, however, were able to enjoy a full-length bath at home until after the end of the First World War. In 1919, in response to an acute shortage of housing, the postwar coalition government passed a housing act which obliged local authorities to survey their housing needs and make good the deficiency with the assistance of a generous government subsidy. The new mandatory council homes built from 1919 were put up according to the recommendations of the Tudor Walters Report of 1918. These embodied a widely held view that new working-class housing should incorporate vastly improved standards of design, comfort and convenience. The report recommended a variety of houses to suit different needs and localities, but all included indoor toilets and baths. The simplest plan had a living room with a range where most of the cooking would be done and a back scullery containing a sink, wash copper and bath, while the best plan included the luxury of an upstairs bathroom. At last, the principle had been established that everyone should have a fixed bath in their home, but for several decades this remained more aspiration than fact. Notwithstanding the clearing of slums in the 1930s and the building of council houses, many working-class families continued to live in older properties that were poorly provided with services. In 1919, roughly 10% of British households lacked a plumbed-in bath but the figure was lower still in poorer industrial districts. In South Wales, for example, only 2.4% of the 26,822 working class homes in the Rhondda had fixed indoor baths in 1920. Private landlords were slow to add bathrooms in older properties and many Victorian terraced houses and rural dwellings were not fitted with baths until the 1950s and 1960s. The 1951 census revealed that 37% of households had no bath at all, not even a shared bath and the 1961 census, the first to ask about hot water taps, showed that 22% of the population still had no hot water tap. There was still a requirement, therefore, for portable baths and whilst the traditional hip bath could still be purchased in the 1920s, galvanised iron baths still featured in hardware catalogues in the mid-1950s.[28]

In the 1920s and 1930s more private houses were built than council houses. New middle-class suburbs, typified by the three-bedroom semi-detached house, but also containing detached houses and bungalows, were developed on the outskirts of most towns and cities. House building reached a boom phase in about 1933/4, and in 1934 the British Bath Maker's Association adopted the slogan: 'A Bath in Every Home', with the aim of attaching the fortunes of the bath manufacturers to the coat-tails of the house builders.[29] Total bath production rose from 199,000 in 1930 to 415,000 in 1934, representing about 85 per cent of the home-market supply; German, French and Hungarian manufacturers also imported baths. By 1935 bath sales for the old established West Bromwich iron founders,

'The only effective way of cleansing the skin is by the free use of water.' Domestic Economy: a Class Book for Girls, 1877.

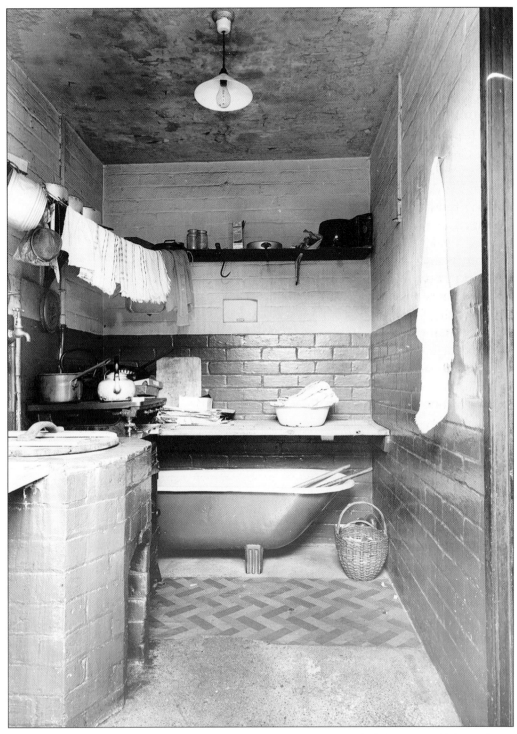

A kitchen on the Penpole Estate, Shirehampton, Bristol, completed at the end of the First World War to house munitions workers. The photograph was taken in the mid-1950s prior to modernisation and shows the basic facilities of the original design with a bath squeezed into a tiny back room, less than 6 ft wide, that also contained a wash copper, Belfast sink and gas cooker. (*Bristol Record Office*)

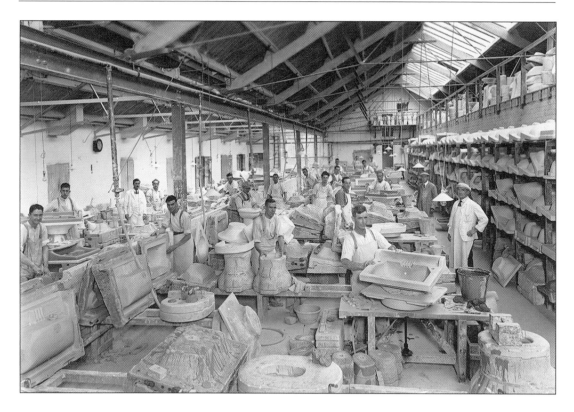

Archibald Kenrick and Sons, accounted for approximately 39 per cent of the company's turnover.[30]

In America, a three-year survey completed in 1928, under the auspices of the General Federation of Women's Clubs, revealed that more than 20 million Americans – roughly 17 per cent of the population – still lived in dwellings without a bathroom. In rural America, where obtaining a car was then a higher priority, the figure was probably higher: 'why, you can't go to town in a bath tub!' declared one rural woman whose family owned a car but not a bath in the 1920s.[31] The leading American sanitaryware manufacturers, however, aimed to stimulate consumer demand for bathroom fittings by introducing new fashionable designs and coloured suites. In December 1927 the Kohler Company of Kohler, Wisconsin, introduced their 'Color Ware' through a full-page colour advertisement in America's most widely read magazine, the *Saturday Evening Post*. Prior to the launch the company had placed samples of coloured fixtures in their showrooms and had been encouraged by the favourable response from the public, especially from women who remarked on the 'striking and beautiful color effects'.[32] The huge Standard Sanitary Manufacturing Co. of Pittsburgh, created by a merger in 1899, soon followed. In 1929 they offered a choice of ten colours with exotic names such as 'St Porchaire brown', 'Clair de Lune blue' and 'Rose du Barry'.

The interior of the sanitary department at Pountneys in Fishponds, Bristol, showing the manufacture of earthenware washbasins, *c.* 1930. (*Bristol City Museum and Art Gallery*)

Coloured bathroom fittings soon reached Britain, where through Hollywood movies, American influence was all-pervasive. In about 1929 Armitage became the first British sanitaryware manufacturer to add a single-colour after-glaze to their products. The colour was sponged on after the first firing. Coloured fittings arrived in Britain just in time to provide the middle-class homeowner with the means of maintaining an element of exclusivity in the bathroom. After a decade of council-house building across the country, fitted bathrooms no longer had an exclusive middle-class image, so the choice of a more expensive coloured suite over the white ones provided in council homes was one way of maintaining the class distinction. Hardware catalogues of the 1930s usually contained colour plates showing *en suite* bathrooms with fittings in a range of colours with wall and floor tiles to match. In 1939 Rowe Brothers of Exeter and Bristol supplied porcelain enamelled cast-iron baths in three shades of green, grey blue, smoke grey, electric blue, primrose, yellow, lavender, pink, and black.[33]

Black was suddenly chic. In America, the architect, Ely Jacques Kahn, selected jet-black Kohler fittings for his bathroom installation at the Metropolitan Museum's annual exhibition of American industrial art in 1929.[34] Chromium also became popular for bathroom fittings such as heated towel rails and taps, and was used with great effect against black. Again, the fashion crossed the Atlantic. In 1933, the artist Paul Nash (1889–1946) designed a bathroom for the London home of Tilly Losch, 35 Wimpole Street, with black fittings, glass wall panels and ceiling mirrors.[35] By 1939 the 'Nuline' range of baths made by A. Hutchison and Son of London could be supplied with black, non-wavy glass panels with decorative border lines.[36] Water closet – or 'toilet' – seats appeared in

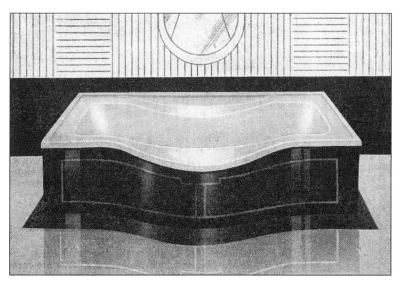

The 'Nuline' bath made by A. Hutchison and Son, Hancock Road, London E3, in 1939. The camber of the front was designed to reflect more light and add lustre to the pastel colours of the panels. This one is shown with a black, non-wavy glass panel inlaid with a steel grey decorative border line.

the 1930s made of bakelite plastic which could be made in colour to match the rest of the bathroom. In 1939 the 'Permax' moulded lavatory seat made by Alfred Goslet and Co., London, was available in black, white and dark walnut, but unlike real wood the polished finish was claimed to be permanent and immune to scratches – an important consideration as women's suspender clips caused scratches in wooden seats.[37] It is a strange observation that the black plastic toilet seat, one of the most basic and utilitarian domestic articles of the mid-twentieth century was born of avant-garde thirties style.

The fashion in the 1930s home was towards simple interior furnishings and fittings. Fewer middle-class families could afford to keep a servant, and anything ornamental that could harbour dust was condemned. So in the bathroom, free-standing, claw-foot bath tubs were now regarded as old fashioned, fussy and inconvenient: sweeping the dust from underneath the bath could, after all, cause respectable housewives to acquire that condition usually associated with servants, 'house maid's knee'. Instead, square-ended baths with panelled sides became popular. Simpler fittings, however, were not necessarily dull. Washbasins appeared in the 'Streamline Moderne' or 'Jazz Modern' style with the same sharp geometric forms found on art deco

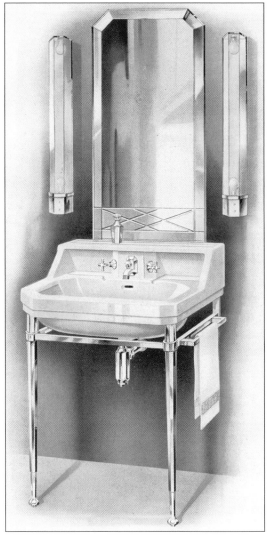

furnishings, radios and the facades of some cinemas. A characteristic feature of thirties baths and basins was the 'cut-corner' of the rim or edge. Supplied in various colours there was just a hint of Hollywood glamour in these 1930s bathroom designs. The films of Cecil B. DeMille (1881–1959), seen by millions of women, featured exotic film stars reclining in bubble baths, epitomising the glamour, beauty and wealth that many wished to bring to their own lives. In the 1920s and 1930s, the principles on which the Victorians had promoted bathing, including the development of robust constitutions and strong characters, diminished in importance as many people, taking their cue from film stars such as Gloria Swanson (1897–1980), were prepared to admit to the sensuous pleasures of bathing.

The 1920s and 1930s saw the widespread adoption of electricity in British homes. Electric lighting could form an important

The 'Rowanco' washbasin of Rowe Brothers, Exeter, was designed in 1930. It has 'cut-corners' to the rim and is flanked by two Art Deco electric wall lights. The basin was made of white 'porcelain enamelled' fireclay and fitted with screw-down taps, a mixing box, central supply nozzle and towel rail stand. The fittings were chromium plated and the unit included the 'brilliant cut and bevelled mirror'.

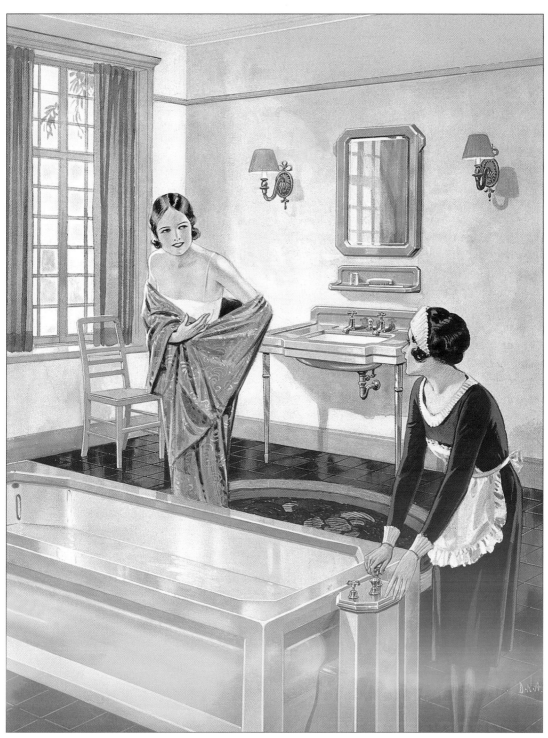

An art-deco bathroom from a Twyford's advertisement, *c.* 1930. Makers took their inspiration from Hollywood films where film producers frequently featured glamorous film stars disrobing in luxurious bathrooms. The room has electric lighting and a 'Moderne'-style rug, while the free-standing bath is enclosed with panelling and has the fashionable 'cut corners' on the rim. (*Twyford Bathrooms*)

component of the overall decorative scheme with art-deco-style wall
lights, for example, fitted above the washbasin: Paul Nash's bespoke
bathroom for Tilly Losch was lit with neon tube lights. Electric wall
heaters also appeared providing an alternative to smelly paraffin
stoves. Bathroom scales and small rectangular stools also became
popular in the 1930s. 'Detecto' bathroom scales, made in the USA,
were sold in Britain in the 1930s: there were eighteen models to
choose from in five different colours, one of which had attracted
orders in America for 60,000 after being exhibited in the 1939
Chicago Fair.[38]

Many bath designs dating from the 1930s continued to be made
until the end of the 1950s when fittings acquired smoother
altogether more rounded lines typified by the bow-fronted basin.
During the 1950s 'vitreous china', a dense, non-porous pottery
originally developed in America which had slowly appeared in
Britain in the 1920s and 1930s, largely replaced earthenware and
fireclay for ceramic bathroom fittings. The impervious body of
vitreous china was formed of various carefully prepared mixtures of
plastic ball clay, china clay and a flux that helps fuse or vitrify the
body. In the biscuit state, the body has a low-water absorption, but
pieces are glazed to avoid staining. Plastic fittings also appeared in
the 1950s and 1960s, although attempts to make taps of plastic were

A fully equipped luxury
bathroom on display at the
Mayfair showrooms of Shanks
and Co., New Bond Street in
1939.

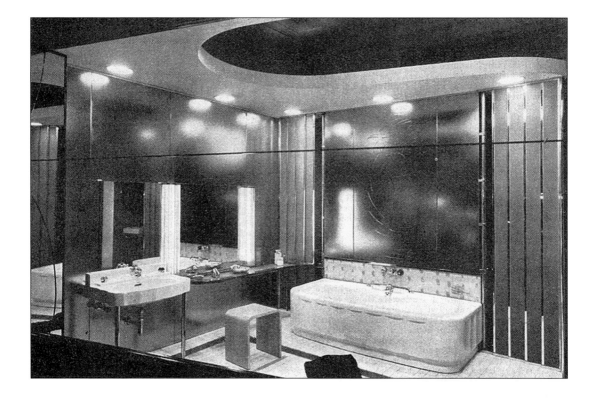

a failure. In the 1950s and 1960s, bathroom decor was influenced by twentieth century 'kitsch', which included specially made bathroom wallpapers printed with sea shells, sea horses and various types of fish. Through a wider choice of accessories and ornaments – large sea shells, for example, brought back from holidays overseas – bathroom interiors became more idiosyncratic and personalised. Children could play in the bath with toys – rubber ducks and plastic boats – specially made for bathtime.

The late 1960s saw the arrival of a new range of colours for bathroom suites. Twyford's 'Pampas' – one of the most popular of all modern bathroom colours – was launched in December 1967, and in April 1979, they withdrew primrose yellow after forty-seven years' continuous production.[39] In 1968 Armitage Ware launched 'avocado' – a dull green – which became enormously popular during the 1970s. Thereafter, and into the 1980s, new names came thick and fast, so that in 1982 Twyford's could offer approaching a dozen colours, including soft brown 'Mink', deep 'Damask' red, and a new shade called 'Almond' which harked back to ivory, popular in the 1880s. Suites were also made by various makers in chocolate brown, deep blue and black. The 1980s also saw a revival of 'traditional' styles by firms such as Heritage Bathrooms. Twyford's introduced their first Victorian-style suite, 'Chantal', in 1995 and two years later, 'Clarice' in the art-deco style. Doulton, meanwhile, introduced their 'nostalgia' range including 'Chelsea', based on a turn of the century design and 'Picasso', an art-deco suite. And then the old firm of Thomas Crapper and Co. was rescued from dormancy and in 1999 launched a water closet, the 'Venerable', along with cisterns and washbasins based on items from the company's late Victorian range. In the 1990s colour fittings were generally less popular and bathroom showrooms were dominated by bathroom suites in white.

In Britain *en suite* bathrooms – that is, reached from within a bedroom – became increasingly common from the 1980s. The idea had originated in America. As early as 1853 the Mount Vernon Hotel at Cape May, a New Jersey resort, had added baths to all its rooms.[40] By the 1920s *en suite* rooms were common in modern American hotels, some having as many as 2,000 bedrooms each with its own bathroom.[41] Additional bathrooms found in late twentieth-century British homes were usually supplied with showers, which were cheaper than baths and took up less space. Ownership of more than one bath remained rare. In October 1999 new building regulations made the installation of a downstairs water closet and washbasin for use by disabled persons compulsory.

A handful of older houses, however, managed to survive .ne twentieth century without ever acquiring a fitted bath or inloor

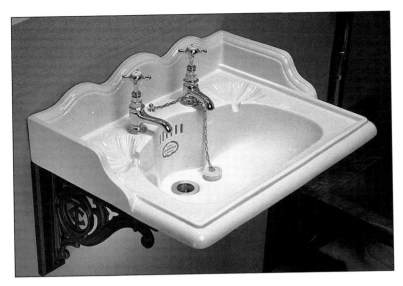

An authentic late Victorian-style lavatory washbasin introduced by Thomas Crapper and Co., Stratford on Avon, in 1999. The only differences to the original are minor alterations to enable connection to modern plumbing and the use of vitreous china in place of earthenware. (*Thomas Crapper and Co. Ltd*)

water closet. One, strangely enough, was next-door-but-one to the author in Bristol. The terraced town house, built in 1893/4, was occupied by a woman in her nineties who had lived there for half a century. She continued to use the water closet in the backyard until a few days before her death in August 2000. She had no bathroom and the water supply did not extend beyond the kitchen. Following her death the house was modernised in early 2001. Hot and cold water was at last extended upstairs and a small back bedroom converted into a bathroom in readiness for new tenants. After all, at the start of the twenty-first century, a bathroom and indoor toilet are two of life's basic necessities.

Select List of Water-Closet Trade Names 1870–1914

Until about 1870 most water-closet names were merely descriptive such as 'Warner's Self-Acting Pan Closet' or 'Jenning's Patent India-Rubber Tube Closet', but shortly after 1870 water closets began to acquire distinctive trade names. Two early ones were the 'Holborn' and 'Universal' closet, made by B. Finch at the Holborn Sanitary Works, London, which had appeared by 1872. Towards the end of the decade the number of names increased as manufacturers doubtless tried to steal an edge on their competitors.

This select list of closet names from the 1870s to 1914 provides some idea of the extraordinary range of names attached to water closets. It does not pretend to be exhaustive and I would be pleased to hear of other names along with the name of the manufacturer and a date. The list also provides some idea of the places of manufacture. Although London and the Staffordshire pottery towns dominate, the list contains closets produced by manufacturers in many other parts of the country. The dates provided for the various models denote the earliest printed record found for that model and not when it is believed – or claimed – to have been introduced. Nevertheless, where the date is beyond all doubt – as with the 'Dolphin', for example, the design of which, was registered on 31 December 1884, the date is in bold.

Some of the names were formally registered according to trademark legislation of the mid-1870s, but some, like the 'Artisan' and 'Waverley', were used by more than one maker for different models. Similarly, some manufacturers used the same name for different types. Thus Doulton and Co. applied the name 'Lambeth' to several different closets over a thirty-year period. A particularly confusing case is George Jennings's wash-out closet. First patented in 1852, it was later known as the 'Monkey' closet, but as this name does not appear until 1884, this is the date listed below and not 1852. Thus the dates relate to the introduction of the name and not necessarily of the model or type. The list, nevertheless, captures something of the spirit of the time, with many famous names present — Twyford's 'Unitas' and 'Deluge', the 'Closet of the Century' by George Jennings and my favourite, the 'Clencher' by James Duckett of Burnley.

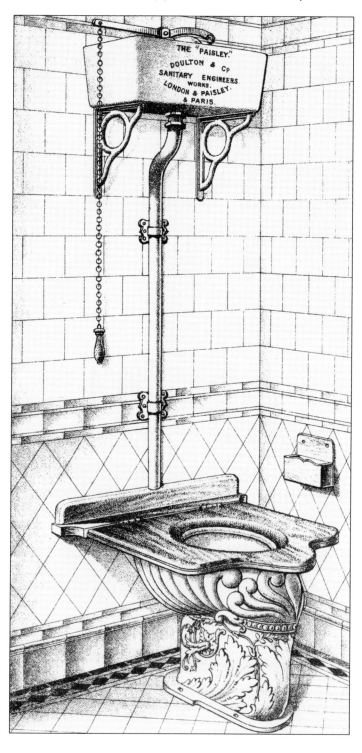

Doulton and Co.'s pedestal 'Combination' wash-out closet with raised acanthus decoration, *c.* 1895. This closet was available in stoneware or glazed fireclay which was marketed as 'White Queensware'. The closet is connected to a cast-iron 'Paisley' cistern made at the company's iron foundry in Paisley, Scotland.

Trade name	Manufacturer/supplier	Date
Alliance (wash-out)	Thomas Twyford, Hanley	1884
Amphora (hopper)	Smeaton and Co., Southwark, London	**1886**
Anchor (wash-down)	Broad and Co., Paddington, London	1910
Argentina (wash-out)	Morrison, Ingram and Co., Manchester	1895
Ariston (wash-down/ slop sink)	Sharpe Bros, Swadlincote	1895
Artisan (basin and trap)	Beard Dent and Hellyer, Strand, London	1877
Artisan (wash-down)	Baxendale and Co., Manchester	1892
Avalanche (wash-out)	J. Warner and Sons, Cripplegate, London	1885
Banner	Sharp and Co., Holborn, London	1884
Barrhead (syphonic)	Shanks and Co., Barrhead	1894
Beaufort (wash-down)	Humpherson and Co., Chelsea, London	1885
Brighton (hopper pan)	George Jennings, Stangate, London	1907
Briton (wash-down)	J. and M. Craig, Kilmarnock	1901
Burton (wash-down)	Sharpe Bros, Swadlincote	1895
Caledon (wash-down)	Sharpe Bros, Swadlincote	1895
Canterbury (wash-down)	George Jennings, Stangate	1907
Cardinal (wash-down)	Thomas Twyford, Hanley	1894
Capstan (wash-down)	Sharpe Bros, Swadlincote	1895
Cascade (wash-out)	Morrison, Ingram and Co., Manchester	1887
Cataract (wash-out)	Sharpe Bros, Swadlincote	1895
Cecebe (wash-out)	Sharpe Bros, Swadlincote	1895
Cedric (wash-down)	Sharpe Bros, Swadlincote	**1891**
Celt (wash-down)	J. and M. Craig, Kilmarnock	1901
Centric (wash-down)	J. and M. Craig, Kilmarnock	1914
Cerus (combined wash-out/valve)	Phillips and Son, London	1886
Chelsea (wash-down)	Thomas Crapper and Co., Chelsea, London	1888
Circe (wash-down)	Sharpe Bros, Swadlincote	1895
Citizen (wash-down)	Shanks and Co., Barrhead	1886
Clencher (wash-down)	J. Duckett and Sons, Burnley	1897
Climax	Smeaton and Sons, London	1889
Climax (tipper closet)	J. Duckett and Sons, Burnley	1914
Closet of the Century (syphonic)	George Jennings, Stangate, London	**1894**
Closet for the Million (pan and trap)	George Jennings, Stangate, London	1872
Colenso (wash-out)	Pountney and Co., Bristol	1906
Colonial (wash-down)	F. Winkle, Stoke-on-Trent	1895
Colossal (wash-down)	Pountney and Co., Bristol	1906
Column (wash-down)	J. Tylor and Sons, Newcastle Street, London	**1890**
Combination (wash-out)	Doulton and Co., Lambeth, London	1884
Combination (wash-down)	Shanks and Co., Barrhead	1886
Compactum (wash-down)	Shanks and Co., Barrhead	
Complete (wash-out)	Charles Winn and Co., Birmingham	1884
Compound (wash-down)	J. Tylor and Sons, Newgate Street, London	1894
Cornbrooke (wash-out)	Morrison, Ingram and Co., Manchester	1895
Crescent (valve)	J. Warner and Son, Cripplegate, London	1884
Crown (wash-out)	Thomas Twyford, Hanley	1882

Trade name	Manufacturer/supplier	Date
Darrah (wash-down)	Baxendale and Co., Manchester	1892
Deap Seal (wash-down)	George Jennings, Stangate, London	1907
Deluge (wash-down)	Thomas Twyford, Hanley	1887
Derby (wash-out)	Sharpe Bros, Swadlincote	1895
Desideratum	Morrison, Ingram and Co., Manchester	1887
Dill (LCC pattern wash-down)	Broad and Co., Paddington, London	1910
Dolphin (wash-out)	J. Dimmock and Co., Hanley	**1884**
Eastwood Sanitary (wash-out)	T. and W. Farmiloe , Westminster, London	1886
Economic (wash-out)	George Jennings, Stangate, London	1894
Empire (wash-down)	Edward Johns, Armitage, Staffordshire	
English Made (wash-out)	John Jones, Chelsea, London	1906
Eos (wash-out)	G. Farmiloe and Sons, St John Street, London	1884
Eos (wash-down)	T. and G. Farmiloe, Westminster, London	1886
Era (valve)	George Jennings, Stangate, London	1907
Esser (wash-down)	Samuel Hunt Rowley, Swadlincote	1898
European (side-outlet valve)	R.F. Dale and Co., Southwark, London	**1884**
Excelsior (wash-out)	Daniel T. Bostel, Brighton	1877
Excelsior (syphonic)	George Jennings, Stangate, London	1907
Excentric (wash-down)	J. and M. Craig, Kilmarnock	1914
Exhibition (valve)	T. and W. Farmiloe, Westminster, London	1884
Federationalist (wash-down)	Sharpe Bros, Swadlincote	1895
Fenelon (wash-out)	Sharpe Bros, Swadlincote	1895
Fleet (wash-down)	Everard and Co., London and Birmingham	1892
Free Flushing (wash-out)	Charles Winn and Co., Birmingham	1884
Gladiator (wash-down)	Cauldon Potteries (Etablisments Porcher)	1905
Grosvenor (valve)	John Bolding and Sons, London	1884
Guardian	Broad and Co., Paddington	1910
Hadfield (wash-down)	Morrison, Ingram and Co., Manchester	1895
Hindustan (Oriental)	Pountney and Co., Bristol	1906
Hindi (Oriental)	Pountney and Co., Bristol	1906
Holborn (valve)	B. Finch, Holborn, London	1872
Household (wash-down)	Sharpe Bros, Swadlincote	1895
Hygate (wash-out)	George Jennings, Stangate, London	1907
Hygienic (wash-down)	Dent and Hellyer, Strand, London	1886
Improved Marlboro (wash-down)	Thomas Crapper and Co., Chelsea, London	1901
Invictas (wash-down)	Johnson Bros, Hanley	**1891**
Ivanhoe (wash-down)	Sharpe Bros, Swadlincote	1895
Ivy Lite (wash-down)	George Howson and Sons, Hanley	1895
Kenon (hopper)	John Bolding and Sons, London	1885
Kent (hopper pan)	George Jennings, Stangate, London	1907
Kenwhar (wash-down)	Thomas Crapper and Co., Chelsea	1915
Lambeth (pan closet)	Doulton and Co., Lambeth, London	1889
Lambeth (trapless)	Doulton and Co., Lambeth, London	1885
Lambeth (wash-out)	Doulton and Co., Lambeth, London	1879
Lambeth (valve)	Doulton and Co., Lambeth, London	1889
Latestas (wash-down)	Johnson Bros, Hanley	1891
Leeds (wash-down)	Joseph Cliff and Sons, Wortley, Leeds	1901
Levern (syphonic)	Shanks and Co., Barrhead	1914

Trade name	Manufacturer/supplier	Date
Lillyman (basin and trap)	Thomas Twyford, Hanley	1879
Lincote (wash-down)	Sharpe Bros, Swadlincote	1895
Liverpool (cottage)	Sharpe Bros, Swadlincote	1895
Liverpool Hopper (cottage)	Shanks and Co, Barrhead	1886
Maelstrom (syphonic)	J. and M. Craig, Kilmarnock	1900
Magna (wash-down)	George Jennings, Stangate, London	1907
Manor (wash-down)	Sharpe Bros, Swadlincote	1895
Marlboro (wash-down)	Thomas Crapper, Chelsea, London	1887
Metropolitan (wash-down)	Baxendale and Co., Manchester	1892
Midland (wash-down)	George Jennings, Stangate, London	1907
Million (wash-down)	J. and M. Craig, Kilmarnock	1901
Modern (wash-down)	Shanks and Co., Barrhead	1914
Monkey (wash-out)	George Jennings, Stangate, London	1884
National (wash-out)	Thomas Twyford, Hanley	1879
Nautilus (hopper)	Smeaton Son and Co., Southwark, London	**1886**
Nelgate (wash-down)	George Jennings, Stangate, London	1907
Nestor (valve)	Henry Conolly, Hampstead, London	1884
Newland (wash-down)	George Jennings, Stangate, London	1907
Newton (wash-down)	George Jennings, Stangate, London	1907
Okeanos (wash-down)	Morrison, Ingram and Co., Manchester	1895
Optimus (valve)	Dent and Hellyer, Strand, London	1884
Orion (wash-down)	Thomas Twyford, Hanley	1898
Ovington (wash-down)	Thomas Crapper and Co., Chelsea, London	1888
Oxford (wash-out)	Dom. Engineering and Sanitary App. Co., London	1884
Paragone (wash-down)	George Jennings, Stangate, London	1907
Parkstone (wash-down)	George Jennings, Stangate, London	1894
Patent Crown (wash-out)	Shanks and Co., Barrhead	1884
Patent Pan (wash-out)	Sharpe Bros, Swadlincote	1884
Pedestal Hygienic (wash-down)	Dent and Hellyer, Strand, London	**1885**
Pedestal Vase (wash-out)	George Jennings, Stangate, London	**1884**
Peel (wash-down)	Broad and Co., Paddington, London	1910
Perfection Darrah's patent (wash-down)	Baxendale and Co., Manchester	1891
Planet (wash-down)	Thomas Twyford, Hanley	1894
Plinius (wash-out)	J. and M. Craig, Kilmarnock	1914
Poole (wash-down)	George Jennings, Stangate, London	1907
Portland (wash-down)	George Jennings, Stangate, London	1907
Praed (wash-down)	Broad and Co., Paddington, London	1910
Primrose (wash-down)	Sharpe Bros, Swadlincote	**1888**
Progress (wash-down)	Perrin, Hughes and Co., Liverpool	
Rapid (tipper closet)	J. Duckett and Son, Burnley	1899
Reading (cottage pan)	Sharpe Bros., Swadlincote	1905
Regent (valve)	Shanks and Co., Barrhead	1914
Repton (wash-out)	Sharpe Bros., Swadlincote	1895
Revolver (wash-down)	Broad and Co., Paddington, London	1910
Ricardia (wash-down)	Edward Johns, Armitage, Staffordshire	1894
Rilcote (wash-down)	Sharpe Bros, Swadlincote	1895
Rivoli (wash-down)	Sharpe Bros, Swadlincote	1895
Rutland (wash-down)	George Jennings, Stangate, London	1907

Trade name	Manufacturer/supplier	Date
Salisbury (wash-down)	George Jennings, Stangate, London	1907
Seal (wash-down)	George Jennings, Stangate, London	1907
Sealon (two-piece wash-down)	Broad and Co., Paddington, London	1910
Sequel (wash-out)	Everard and Co., London and Birmingham	1892
Severn (wash-out)	Sharpe Bros, Swadlincote	1895
Shanks Patent Syphonic Closet	Shanks and Co., Barrhead	1891
Sharcote (wash-down)	Sharpe Bros, Swadlincote	1905
Shrewsbury Tipper (hopper)	Thomas Gregory, Clapham, London	1884
Simplex (valve)	T. and W. Farmiloe, Westminster, London	1884
Simplicitas (wash-down)	Doulton and Co., Lambeth, London	1897
Sirex (two-piece wash-down)	Broad and Co., Paddington, London	1910
Smethwick (wash-out)	Everard and Co., London and Birmingham	1892
Soil Hide (wash-down)	Sharpe Bros, Swadlincote	1895
Solgate (wash-down)	George Jennings, Stangate, London	1907
Spate	Morrison, Ingram and Co., Manchester	1895
Special (valve)	John Warner and Sons, Cripplegate, London	1884
Speedwell (wash-down)	Doulton and Co., Lambeth, London	1906
Stangate (wash-down)	George Jennings, Stangate, London	1907
Subitus (wash-down)	Gardiner and Sons, Ironmongers, Bristol	*c.* 1894
Sussex (wash-down)	Everard and Co., London and Birmingham	1892
Swanton (wash-down)	Sharpe Bros, Swadlincote	1895
Swiftor (wash-down)	Broad and Co., Paddington, London	1910
Times (wash-out)	Shanks and Co., Barrhead	1886
Togo (wash-down)	Pountney and Sons, Bristol	1906
Tornado (wash-out)	Thomas Twyford, Hanley	1889
Torrent	J.G. Slider and Co., Southwark, London	1884
Torrentia (syphonic)	J. and M. Craig, Kilmarnock	1914
Trefoil (wash-down)	Joseph Cliff and Sons, Wortley, Leeds	1901
Trent (wash-down)	Johnson Brothers, Hanley	1894
Trident (wash-down)	Thomas Twyford, Hanley	1894
Trinal (wash-out)	Morrison, Ingram and Co., Manchester	1887
Triple Alliance (wash-down)	Freeman Bros, Battersea, London	1895
Triton (wash-down)	Morrison, Ingram and Co., Manchester	1890
Triune (wash-down)	Samuel Hunt Rowley, Swadlincote	1898
Tubal (wash-out)	Shanks and Co., Barrhead	1884
Twin Basin (plug)	Capper and Son, Fenchurch Street, London	1884
Twycliffe (syphonic)	Thomas Twyford, Hanley	**1894**
Tylerox (wash-down)	Hayward-Tylor and Co., London	1896
Ultimatum (trapless)	J.G. Stidder and Co., Southwark, London	1884
Undine (wash-out)	Thomas Twyford, Hanley	1894
Unitas (wash-out)	Thomas Twyford, Hanley	**1882**
United Kingdom (syphonic)	Baxendale and Co., Manchester	1896
Universal	B. Finch, Holborn, London	1872
Universal (valve)	J.G. Stidder and Co., Southwark, London	1884
Utilis (wash-down)	Sharpe Bros, Swadlincote	1895
Utility (basin and trap)	George Jennings, Stangate, London	1907
Validus (wash-down)	George Howson and Sons, Hanley	**1894**
Vauxhall (cottage)	Everard and Co., London and Birmingham	1892

Trade name	Manufacturer/supplier	Date
Velos (wash-out)	Thomas Twyford, Hanley	1894
Victoria (wash-out)	Sharpe Bros, Swadlincote	1895
Victor (wash-out)	Sharpe Bros, Swadlincote	1895
Villa (valve)	John Warner and Sons, Cripplegate, London	1884
Vortex (one-piece closet and trap)	Beard, Dent and Hellyer, Strand, London	1879
Vyrnwy (wash-down)	Thomas Twyford, Hanley	1889
Warwick (wash-down)	J. Tylor and Sons, Newgate Street, London	1894
Washago (wash-down)	Sharpe Bros, Swadlincote	1895
Wash-out (wash-out)	James Woodward, Swadlincote	**1878**
Water-battery (wash-out)	Dent and Hellyer, Strand, London	1891
Wave (wash-out)	Sharpe Bros, Swadlincote	1895
Waveonic (wash-down)	Morrison, Ingram and Co., Manchester	1895
Waverley (wash-down)	Sharpe Bros, Swadlincote	1895
Waverley (wash-down)	Sherwin and Cotton, Hanley	1895
Waverley (wash-down)	Doulton and Co., Lambeth, London	1903
Windsor (wash-out)	Sharpe Bros, Swadlincote	1895
Wingate (wash-out)	George Jennings, Stangate, London	1907
Zetland (wash-down)	George Jennings, Stangate, London	1907
Zone (wash-down)	Thomas Twyford, Hanley	1894

Places to Visit

Abbey Pumping Station, off Abbey Lane, Leicester, LE4 5PX.

Beamish, North of England Open Air Museum, County Durham, DH9 0RG.

Blaise Castle House Museum, Henbury, Bristol, BS10 7QS.

Castle Drogo, Drewsteignton, nr Exeter, Devon EX6 6PB.

Crossness Engines, The Old Works, Crossness Sewage Treatment Works, Belvedere Road, Abbey Wood, London, SE2 9AQ (visits by appointment two days a month).

Dorset County Museum, High Street West, Dorchester, DT1 1XA.

Georgian House Museum, 7 Great George Street, Bristol, BS1 5PR.

Gladstone Pottery Museum, Uttoxeter Road, Longton, Stoke-on-Trent, ST3 1PQ.

Heritage and Arts Resource Centre, Swadlincote, Derbyshire (due to open 2003).

Mr Straw's House, 7 Blyth Grove, Worksop, Nottinghamshire, S81 0JE.

Museum in the Park, Mansion House, Stratford Park, Stratford Road, Stroud, Gloucestershire, GL5 4AF.

Museum of Liverpool Life, Pier Head, Liverpool, L3 1PZ.

Museum of Welsh Life, St Fagans, Cardiff, CF5 6XB.

Port Sunlight Heritage Centre, 95 Greendale Road, Port Sunlight, Wirral, Merseyside, CH62 4XE.

Russell-Cotes Art Gallery and Museum, East Cliff, Bournemouth, Dorset, BH1 3AA.

Science Museum, Exhibition Road, South Kensington, London, SW7 2DD.

Spode Museum, Church Street, Stoke-on-Trent, ST4 1BX.

The Tenement House, 145 Buccleuch Street, Garnethill, Glasgow G3 6QN.

Town House Museum of Lynn Life, 46 Queen Street, King's Lynn, Norfolk, PE30 5DQ.

Tredegar House, Coed Kernew, Newport, Gwent, NP10 8YW.

Twyford Bathrooms, Lawton Road, Alsager, Stoke-on-Trent, ST7 2DF (visits by appointment).

Wimpole Hall, Arrington, Royston, Cambridgeshire, SG8 0BW.

Notes

Chapter One

1. C. Morris, *Craft, Industry and Everyday Life: Wood and Woodworking in Anglo-Scandinavian and Medieval York*, York Archaeological Trust, 2000, pp. 2304–8 and *Yorvik the Viking City*, p. 14.
2. A.J. Taylor, *Conway Castle and Town Walls*, HMSO, 1957 and 1966, p. 13.
3. The National Trust, *Little Moreton Hall*, 1995 and 1998, p. 22.
4. Sir John Vanbrugh's Designs for Kings Weston, Bristol Record Office, BRO 33746.
5. L. Lambton, *Temples of Convenience*, Pavillion, 1995, p. 40.
6. 'The Hardwick Hall Inventory of 1601', *Furniture History*, 1971, pp. 16, 32.
7. J. Cox and B. Trinder, *Yeomen and Colliers in Telford*, Phillimore, 1980, p. 24.
8. F.W. Steer, *Farm and Cottage Inventories of Mid-Essex, 1635–1749*, Essex Record Office, 1950.
9. Cox and Trinder, p. 268.
10. R. Latham and W. Mathews, *The Diary of Samuel Pepys*, Bell and Hyman, London, 1972, vol. 6, p. 244.
11. *The Letters and Journals of Lady Mary Coke*, Edinburgh, 1889, vol. 2, p. 102.
12. François de la Rochefoucauld, *A Frenchman's Year in Suffolk*, 1784 ed., trans. by Norman Scarfe,

Suffolk Record Society, vol. XXX, 1988, p. 23.
13. H. Austin, *A Report on the Sanatory [sic] Condition of Worcester*, T. Eaton, Worcester, 1847, p. 4. The following year Austin became secretary of the new Board of Health.
14. *Ibid.*
15. See, for example, the satirical print attributed to William Hogarth, *Sawney in the Bog House*, 17 June 1745 (British Museum, Prints and Drawings, PS 133064).
16. F. Thompson, *Lark Rise to Candleford*, 1945, p. 263.
17. C. Sale, *The Specialist*, Specialist Publishing Co., St Louis, Minnesota, 1929 and Putnam and Co., London, 1929.
18. W.G. Savage, *Rural Housing*, 1915, p. 63.
19. E. Grey, *Cottage Life in a Hertfordshire Village*, Fisher Knight and Co. Ltd, St Albans, 1934, p. 51.
20. Annual Report for 1912 of the Medical Officer of Health for Cornwall, cited in Savage, p. 63.
21. Austin, p. 4.
22. Thompson, p. 23.
23. F.G. Heath, *Peasant Life in the West of England*, Sampson Low, Marston Searle and Rivington, London, 1881, p. 113.
24. Evidence of Dr William Budd, House of Commons Parliamentary Papers, 1845, vol. 18, Report of

Sir Henry de la Beche.

25. H. Mayhew, *London Labour and the London Poor*, Griffin, London, 1851, pp. 495–6.

26. G. Wilson, *A Handbook of Hygiene*, 1873, p. 227.

27. *Ibid.,* p. 225.

28. R. Latham and W. Mathews, *The Diary of Samuel Pepys*, vol. 1, p. 269.

29. Mayhew, p. 510.

30. *Ibid.*

31. *Ibid.*

32. *Ibid.*, p. 512.

33. *Ibid.*, p. 509.

34. H. Gavin, *Sanitary Ramblings*, 1848, pp. 47, 56.

35. A. Young, *General View of the Agriculture of Hertfordshire*, 1804, David and Charles, 1971, p. 171. In the early 1840s, the *Hampshire Chronicle* recorded the arrival of nightsoil barges from London in Southampton Water.

36. Mayhew, p. 509.

37. Report of G.T. Clark to the General Board of Health on the Sanitary Condition of Bristol, 1850, p. 104.

38. Grey, p. 51.

39. Wilson, p. 224.

40. R.A. Lewis, *Edwin Chadwick and the Public Health Movement 1832–1854*, 1952, p. 87.

41. Gavin, pp. 13, 18.

42. Mayhew, p. 492.

43. *The Times*, 5 July 1849.

44. S. Halliday, *The Great Stink of London*, 1999, Sutton, Stroud, p. 50.

45. I am indebted to Dr Sally Sheard, Department of Public Health and School of History, Liverpool University, for this information.

46. David Large and Frances Round, *Public Health in Mid-Victorian Bristol*, Bristol Branch of the Historical Association, 1974, pp. 1–9.

47. The Public Health Act, 1875, pt 3, cl. 36.

48. Cottage Sanitation, *JRASE*, 3rd series, vol. 3, 1892, p. 640.

49. See, for example, by-laws made by the Rural District Council of Barton Regis [Gloucestershire], Bristol, 1902 (Bristol Record Office).

50. Savage, p. 61.

Chapter Two

1. See Adam Hart-Davis's discussion of this in *Thunder, Flush and Thomas Crapper*, 1997, p. 46.

2. J.A. Surrey, volume ii, p. 160, quoted in Hellyer, p. 192.

3. J. Ayres, *Building the Georgian City*, Yale, 1998, p. 182.

4. F. Thompson, *History of Chatsworth*, London, p. 73 ff. quoted in Mark Girouard, *The English Country House*.

5. C. Fiennes, *The Illustrated Journeys of Celia Fiennes c. 1682–1712*, ed. Christopher Morris, Macdonald, London, 1984, p. 243.

6. Ayres, pp. 182–3.

7. D. Cruickshank and N. Burton, *Life in the Georgian City*, Viking, 1990, p. 96, *Survey of London*, vol. 39, App. 2.

8. P. Thornton, *Authentic Décor: The Domestic Interior 1620–1920*, 1984, pp. 114–15.

9. R. Campbell, *The London Tradesman*, T. Gardner, 1747, David and Charles, 1969, p. 190.

10. Patent 1775/1105, A. Cummings, p. 2.

11. S. Smiles, *Industrial Biography, Iron Workers and Tool Makers*, John Murray, London 1863, p. 185.

12. Patent 1778/1177, J. Bramah, p. 1.

13. J. Woodforde, *The Diary of a Country Parson 1758–1802*, Oxford University Press, 1978, p. 116, and *Gilbert White's Year*, Oxford University Press, 1982, p. 18.

14. H.W. Dickinson, *Joseph Bramah and His Inventions*, Transactions of

the Newcomen Society, vol. 22, 1942, p. 171.

15. *Ibid.*

16. Invoice from Joseph Bramah to Thomas Anson, 1793 (Staffordshire Record Office D615/E(H)2/1–2). I am indebted to Pamela Sambrook for bringing this to my attention.

17. Patent 1777/1160, L. Prosser.

18. Patent 1796/2111, W. Law.

19. This pan closet was presented to the Science Museum by His Majesty's Office of Works in 1927 having being discovered when the palace was being 'redrained'. The appliance has a lead container and copper pan, Science Museum no. 1927–244.

20. J. Burnett, *A Social History of Housing*, pp. 12–16.

21. Auction particulars, Walcot House (Bath Reference Library).

22. J. Jennings, *The Family Cyclopaedia*, 1821, p. 1,301.

23. H. Mayhew, *London Labour and the London Poor*, p. 496.

24. S. Stevens Hellyer, *Principles and Practices of Plumbing*, 1891, p. 198.

25. Mayhew, *London Labour*, 1861, p. 492.

26. Patent 1855/2047, E. Sharpe.

27. J.H. Walsh, *A Manual of Domestic Economy*, 1857, p. 59.

28. *The Builder*, 1 November 1879, p. 1,198.

29. W. Eassie, *Healthy Houses*, 1872, p. 74, J. Bailey Denton, *Sanitary Engineering*, 1877, p. 73.

30. S. Stevens Hellyer, p. 200.

31. *The Builder*, 1 November 1879, p. 1,198.

32. *Minute Book*, Leicester Highways and Sewerage Committee, 13 August 1849, quoted in J. Spavold, *The Sanitary Pottery Industries of South Derbyshire, 1840–1914*, p. 42.

33. Mayhew, p. 493.

34. H. Austin, *A Report on the Sanatory [sic] Condition of Worcester*, T. Eaton, Worcester, 1847, p. 4.

35. House of Commons Parliamentary Papers, 1845, vol. 18, Report of Sir Henry de la Beche.

36. Parliamentary Papers, 1844, vol. 17, q. 5,891, evidence of Joseph Quick, cited in Halliday, *The Great Stink of London*, p. 34.

37. D. Large and F. Round, *Public Health in Mid-Victorian Bristol*, Bristol Branch of the Historical Association, 1974, p. 12, and J. Latimer, *Annals of Bristol*, vol. 3, 1887, p. 314.

38. I am grateful to Dr Sally Sheard at Liverpool University for this information.

39. Large and Round, pp. 6–7.

40. *The Builder*, 24 October 1885, p. 566.

41. Halliday, ch. 4.

42. *Ibid.*, p. 7.

43. G. Wilson, *Sanitary Hygiene*, 1873, p. 244.

44. Revd C. Girdlestone, *Letters on the Unhealthy Condition of the Lower Class of Dwellings especially in Large Towns*, Longman, London, 1845, p. 69.

45. J.C. Loudon, *Cottage Farm and Villa Architecture*, 1846 ed., p. 243, fig. 437.

46. Girdlestone, p. 69.

47. For example, the 1856 catalogue of John Warner shows enamelled cast-iron hoppers, pp. 50–2 (Science Museum Library).

48. Girdlestone, p. 70.

49. *Ibid.*

50. *The Ironmonger*, 15 March 1884, p. 3.

51. J. Bailey Denton, pp. 73–4 and J.H. Walsh, p. 62.

52. S. Stevens Hellyer, p. 206.

53. Hopper closets are featured in the 1910 catalogue of Broad and Co., Paddington.

54. J.C. Morton, *A Cyclopedia of Agriculture*, Blackie and Son, 1855, p. 560.

55. John Warner and Sons, Catalogue, 1856, p. 43.

56. Wilson, pp. 245–6.

57. *Ibid.*, p. 237.

58. Denton, p. 253.

59. *The Builder*, 19 October 1878, p. 1087.

Chapter Three

1. Quoted in 'The Utilisation of Sewage', *The Ironmonger*, 30 May 1863, p. 127.
2. *Ibid.*
3. H. Mayhew, *London Labour and the London Poor*, 1851, p. 438.
4. R.D. Brigden, *Victorian Farms*, 1986, p. 214.
5. Quoted in *The Builder*, 8 September 1862, p. 800.
6. P.H. Frere, 'The Money Value of Night Soil and of Other Manures', *JRASE*, vol. 24, 1863, p. 127.
7. Brigden, pp. 215–16.
8. S. Halliday, *The Great Stink of London*, Sutton, 1999, p. 116. Halliday provides an account of this debate and how it affected London in his chapter, 'Where there's Muck there's Brass?'
9. *Ibid.*, p.116.
10. *Ibid.*, pp.115–19.
11. Brigden, pp. 217–19.
12. *The Ironmonger*, 30 May 1863, p. 127.
13. H. Moule, 'Earth versus Water for the Removal and Utilisation of Excrementitious Matter', *JRASE*, vol. 24, 1863, p. 112.
14. *Ibid.*, pp. 112–13.
15. G. Wilson, *A Handbook of Hygiene*, 1873, p. 235.
16. *Ibid.*, pp. 113–14.
17. *Ibid.*, p. 114.
18. *Catalogue of Plumbers' Sundries*, Llewellins and James, 1889, p. 380 (Blaise Castle House Museum, Bristol).
19. *The Ironmonger*, 1 September 1873, advertisements.
20. Patent 1873/1867, H. Moule and J.W. Girdlestone.
21. *JRASE*, vol. 24, 1863, p. 116.
22. Dr Augustus Voelcker, 'On the Composition and Agricultural Value of Earth Closet Manure', *JRASE*, vol. 8, 2nd series, 1872, pp. 190–2.
23. M.A. Havinden, *Estate Villages: A Study of the Berkshire Villages of Ardington and East Lockinge*, Lund Humphries, 1966, p. 96.
24. J. Bailey Denton, *Sanitary Engineering*, 1876, p. 222.
25. *JRASE*, vol. 24, 1863, p. 123.
26. *Ibid.*, p. 111.
27. *Ibid.*, pp. 116–17.
28. *Ibid.*, p. 117.
29. Patent 1857/1793, John Lloyd.
30. W. Eassie, *Healthy Houses*, 1872, p. 94.
31. *The Ironmonger*, 6 December 1884, p. 721.
32. Wilson, *A Handbook of Hygiene*, 1873, pp. 227–9.
33. *Ibid.*, p. 229.
34. Patent 1859/648, J.S. Dawes.
35. *The Ironmonger*, 6 December 1884, p. 721.
36. Patent 1866/2988, J.C. Morrell.
37. *The Builder*, 14 June 1884, p. 881 and 26 September 1885, p. 423.
38. J. Bailey Denton, pp. 223–4.
39. J. Bailey Denton, p. 219.
40. G. Wilson, p. 230.
41. J. Bailey Denton, p. 226.
42. *The Builder*, 1 June 1878, p. 556.
43. J. Bailey Denton, pp. 220–1.
44. *The Builder*, 1 June 1878, pp. 555–6.
45. Patent 1868/566, P.N. Goux.
46. J. Bailey Denton, p. 221.
47. *Ibid.*
48. Wilson, p. 231.
49. Savage, p. 61.
50. *House Drainage*, International Corresponding Schools, 1905, p. 2.
51. Voelcker, p. 188.
52. *Ibid.*, p. 190.
53. *The Ironmonger*, 30 May 1863, p. 127.
54. *The Ironmonger*, 29 April 1871, p. 353.
55. *JRASE*, vol. 24, 1863, p. 123.
56. Voelcker, p. 188.
57. Sandwich District Council, Kent, continued to collect buckets, replacing them with empty ones until about 1967. Information supplied to the author by Mrs D. McCabe.
58. Moule's patent earth closets (costing 82s) are included in the 1932 catalogue of the Metal Agencies Company, Bristol, p. 321.

Chapter Four

1. J. Hogg, *London As It Is*, 1837, p. 251.
2. C. Kingsley, *The Water Babies*, 1863 and Macmillan 1885, pp. 29–31.
3. Webster, T., *An Encyclopaedia of Domestic Economy*, Longman, 1844, p. 1,216.
4. R. Latham and W. Mathews, *The Diary of Samuel Pepys*, G. Bell and Sons, 1972, vol. 6, p. 40, 21 February 1664–5.
5. J. Cox and B. Trinder, *Yeomen and Colliers in Telford*, Phillimore, 1980, p. 359.
6. Pinney papers, letter book 2 (Bristol University Library).
7. J.C. Loudon, *Cottage Farm and Villa Architecture*, Longman, 1833, p. 1264.
8. J. Jennings, *Family Cyclopaedia*, 1821, pp. 97–105.
9. *Ibid.*, p. 317.
10. Webster, p. 1216.
11. *Ibid.*, p. 1220.
12. J.H. Walsh, 1857, p. 680.
13. House of Commons Parliamentary Papers, 1845, vol. xviii, Report of Sir Henry de la Beche.
14. *Cassell's Household Guide*, *c.* 1869, p. 46.
15. *The Ironmonger*, 30 May 1863, advertisements. Loveridge had patented the hollow rim in 1856, patent 1856/470.
16. *The Ironmonger*, 1 April 1873, p. 397.
17. The Spode Museum, Stoke-on-Trent, has a blue and white earthenware leg bath, 17¼ in high, in 'Lange Lijsen' pattern, 1820.
18. W. and R. Chambers, *Cookery and Domestic Economy for Young Housewives Including Directions for Servants by the Mistress of a Family*, Edinburgh, 1845, p. 117.
19. Blaise Castle House Museum, Bristol.
20. *Martineau and Smith's Hardware Trade Journal*, 28 February 1882, p. xliii.
21. *Martineau and Smith's Hardware Trade Journal*, 30 June 1882, p. 222.
22. F. Thompson, *Lark Rise to Candleford*, 1945, p. 431.
23. Shower bath, plate from poetical sketches of Scarborough, engraved by Joseph Constantine Stadler (fl. 1780–1812), pub. 1813.
24. John Warner and Sons, brass founders, catalogue, 1856, pp. 146–7 (Science Museum Library).
25. *How We Build*, Sidney Flavel and Co., Leamington Spa, n.d., *c.* 1937, p. 12 (Leamington Spa Public Library).
26. *The Ironmonger*, 30 June 1863, advertisements.
27. Webster, p. 1219.
28. Mrs Caddy, *Household Organisation*, Chapman and Hall, London, 1877, p. 169.
29. The first patent for a kitchen-range boiler was taken out by Joseph Langmead in 1783, patent 1361.
30. *The Ironmonger*, 1861.
31. Patent 1849/12,504, N. Defries. See also the Official Descriptive Catalogue of the Great Exhibition, 1851, vol. II, p. 649.
32. Walsh, pp. 64, 679.
33. Report by the Jurors, The Royal Commission, William Clowes and Son, 1852.
34. *The Ironmonger*, 1 October 1873, p. 1156.
35. Patent 1868/3917, B.W. Maughan. Maughan's original geyser was presented to the Science Museum by the Parkinson Stove Co. in 1913, Science Museum no. 1913–77.
36. *The Ironmonger*, 1 January 1874, p. 35.
37. *Martineau and Smith's Hardware Trade Journal*, 30 April 1880, p. 143.
38. Information provided by letter to the author.
39. *Slater's Directory*, 1850, p. 33.

40. John Warner and Sons, brass
    founders, catalogue, 1856,
    pp. 136–9 for various back-boiler
    arrangements (Science Museum
    Library).
41. Walsh, p. 21.
42. F. Dye, a heating engineer, claimed
    to have coined the term to
    distinguish it from the later
    cylinder system which he described
    as being a recent development in
    1893. *The Ironmonger*, 5 August
    1893, p. 229.
43. *The Ironmonger*, 18 January 1879,
    p. 71.

44. Circulating cylinders and
    systems are included in the
    catalogue of Llewellins and James,
    brass founders of Bristol, 1889,
    pp. 442, 446, but according to
    A.C. Martin, tank systems were
    still being installed in the 1920s.
    Ch. by A.C. Martin, 'Sanitary
    Plumbing and Waste Disposal
    Work', in Harry Newbold Bryant,
    House and Cottage Construction,
    Caxton, London, n.d., *c.* 1930,
    p. 133.

Chapter Five

1. H. Taine, *Notes from England*, 1871,
   pp. 182–3.
2. H.R. Jennings, *Our Homes and How
   to Beautify Them*, 1902, p. 236.
3. P. Thornton, pp. 18, 48.
4. *Ibid.*, p. 188.
5. J.C. Loudon, *Cottage, Farm and
   Villa Architecture*, 1833, p. 1264.
6. T. Webster, 1844, p. 219.
7. Walsh, 1857, p. 679.
8. R. Kerr, *The English Gentleman's
   Household*, 1864, p. 167.
9. *The Builder*, 1 November 1879,
   p. 1217.
10. J. Burnett, *A Social History of
    Housing 1815–1970*, 1978, p. 202.
11. *The Builder*, 1 November 1879,
    p. 1198.
12. G. and W. Grossmith, *The Diary of
    a Nobody*, 1892, Penguin, 1945,
    pp. 42–6.
13. A. Forty, *Objects of Desire*, 1986,
    p. 159.
14. Muthesius, *The English House*,
    1904/5 and 1979, p. 235.
15. See, for example, the 1889
    catalogue of Llewellins and James,
    Bristol, p. 462.
16. *Ibid.*, 21 June 1884, p. 916.
17. *The Builder*, 7 June 1884, p. 847.
18. Supplement to *The Ironmonger*,
    5 October 1889, p. lxxi.
19. Françoise de Bonneville, *The Book
    of the Bath*, trans. Jane Brenton,

Thames and Hudson, London,
1998.
20. P. Thornton, p. 308.
21. J.L. Mott Iron Works, *Illustrated
    Catalogue of Victorian Plumbing
    Fixtures for Bathrooms and Kitchens*,
    New York, 1888, Dover
    Publications, New York, 1987,
    p. 5.
22. J. Barnard, *Victorian Ceramic Tiles*,
    1972, p. 33.
23. Eastlake, 1868 and 1969, Dover
    Publications, New York, p. 50.
24. Lucinda Lambton illustrates a
    bathroom in Cheshire at Pownall
    Hall school which contains de
    Morgan tiles, p. 137.
25. *The Builder*, 18 July 1885, p. 86.
26. Mark Girouard, p. 297.
27. G. White, *Tramways to the Stars,
    George White of Bristol*, Redcliffe,
    1995, p. 35, and information
    kindly provided by Sir George
    White.
28. Doulton and Co., *Catalogue of
    Sanitary Appliances*, 1904, p. 3
    (Science Museum Library).
29. *Mr Straw's House*, The National
    Trust, 1993, pp. 16–17.
30. *Martineau and Smith's Hardware
    Trade Journal*, 30 September 1884,
    advertisement.
31. Muthesius, p. 237.

Chapter Six

1. *The Ironmonger*, September 1886.
2. *The Ironmonger*, 23 August 1884, p. 263.
3. See, for example, the advertisement for the 'Empress' steel bath by Frederick Braby in *The Ironmonger*, 13 September 1884, p. 347.
4. *Gore's Directory of Liverpool*, Mawdesley and Sons, Liverpool, 1859, advertisements, p. 8.
5. Catalogue of Milton, Falkirk and Glasgow, *c.* 1906, p. 999.
6. *The Ironmonger*, 20 July 1878, p. 18.
7. S. Timmins, *Birmingham and the Midland Hardware District*, 1866. pp. 106, 643.
8. *Catalogue of Fitted Sanitary Appliances*, Doulton and Co., 1904, introduction. Porcelain enamel and vitreous enamel were the same thing. Today in Britain, 'vitreous' is generally used while the Americans call it 'porcelain'. I am grateful to Simon Kirby for clarifying this point.
9. *Martineau and Smith's Hardware Trade Journal*, 1 July 1897, p. 10.
10. G.M. Shanks, *The First Hundred Years*, Shanks, 1951, pp. 1–6.
11. 'The Engineering Industries of Manchester', reprinted from *The Ironmonger*, 3 and 10 September 1887, pp. 43–4 and Gilbert M. Shanks, p. 7.
12. P. Atterbury and L. Irvine, *The Doulton Story*, 1979, p. 58.
13. *The Builder*, 9 January 1886, p. 71.
14. Muthesius, 1904/5, p. 236.
15. Shanks were advertising rolled-edge baths in *The Ironmonger* by 1888, *The Ironmonger*, 14 April 1888, p. 5.
16. These prices are taken from *The Victorian House Catalogue*, a reprint of the catalogue of Young and Martin, builders' merchants, Stratford, *c.* 1895, reprinted by Sidgwick and Jackson, 1990.
17. Catalogue of the International Exhibition 1862, p. 45 and patent 1849/12,866, F.T. Rufford.
18. J.L. Mott Iron Works, *Illustrated Catalogue of Victorian Plumbing Fixtures for Bathrooms and Kitchens*, 1888, and Dover Publications, p. 14.
19. J. Hatton, *Twyfords: A Chapter in the History of Pottery*, *c.* 1898, p. 256.
20. Doulton and Co., *Catalogue of Fitted Sanitary Appliances*, 1904, p. 3.
21. Muthesius, p. 236.
22. Patent 1874/1028, W. Smeaton and W.H. Tylor, 1874. In an advertisement for the 'Imperial' bath in 1890, Smeaton's claimed to be the 'original inventor of combination spray baths', R.O. Allsop, *The Turkish Bath*, Spon, London, 1890, p. 4.
23. *The Ironmonger*, 19 October 1878, p. 11.
24. S. Stevens Hellyer, *Principles and Practices of Plumbing*, 1891, p. 248.
25. *The Ironmonger*, 18 September 1886, p. 469.
26. *The Builder*, 21 June 1884, p. 917.
27. This model was also exhibited at the Edinburgh International Exhibition in 1886.
28. *The Ironmonger*, 7 April 1888, p. xlix.
29. Hellyer, p. 248.
30. Allsop, pp. 2 and 5.
31. Doulton catalogue, 1904, p. 3 (Science Museum Library).
32. See, for example, *Sanitary Fittings, International Corresponding Schools*, 1905, p. 37.
33. L. Wright, *Clean and Decent*, p. 115.
34. Warner catalogue, 1856, p. 64, includes two iron washbasins.
35. *The Ironmonger*, 19 October 1878, supplement.
36. Introduced by 1891, Hellyer, p. 244.
37. *The Ironmonger*, 10 May 1890.
38. *Ibid.*, 5 July 1884, p. 15.
39. Timmins, p. 285.
40. *Ibid.*, p. 288. The Rotherham brass

founders, Guest and Chrimes, are
credited with introducing the
screw-down compression tap by
Timmins.

41. *Martineau and Smith's Hardware
    Trade Journal*, 30 July 1881,
    supplement.

42. Llewellins and James, catalogue,
    1889, pp. 471, 499 (Blaise Castle
    House Museum, Bristol).

43. Patent 1877/2056, J. Shanks.

44. Morrison's patent no. 1574,
    advertised in *The Ironmonger*,

10 July 1886, p. xxxvii, and
Abridgements of Patents 1877–83,
pp. 110–11.

45. *Sanitary Fittings*, ICS Reference
    Library, 1905, p. 33.

46. Spong and Co., Manufacturers of
    Domestic Machinery, *Catalogue*,
    n.d., *c.* 1895.

47. *The Ironmonger*, 14 December 1895,
    p. xix.

48. Shanks and Co., *Catalogue of
    Sanitary Appliances*, April 1886,
    p. 1.

Chapter Seven

1. C.R. Fay, *Palace of Industry*,
   Cambridge University Press, 1951,
   p. 76.

2. No evidence, however, has come to
   light to attribute the origin of this
   euphemism specifically to the
   Great Exhibition.

3. Jennings was awarded a prize at the
   Great Exhibition for a water closet,
   although it may have been the india-
   rubber tube closet which impressed
   the jurors. Catalogue no. 810 in class
   XXII, *Exhibition of the Works of
   Industry of All Nations 1851, Reports
   by the Juries*, Royal Commission,
   London, 1852, p. 505.

4. The use of the india-rubber tube
   closets in the superior refreshments
   court is recorded in the *Official
   Descriptive and Illustrated Catalogue
   of the Great Exhibition*, William
   Clowes and Sons, London, 1851,
   vol. II, p. 670. The use of the wash-
   out closet at the exhibition is
   mentioned in George Jennings's
   catalogue of *c.* 1894, p. 33.

5. Patent 1852/14,273. The claim
   that Jennings had introduced his
   closet before the Great Exhibition
   was made in a company catalogue
   of *c.* 1894.

6. Patent 1856/2788.

7. Patents 1858/1500 and 1858/1504.
   However, in 1894 the company
   claimed to have introduced this
   closet in 1862, George Jennings's
   catalogue, 1894, p. 24.

8. G.M. Shanks, *Shanks: The First
   Hundred Years*, 1951, p. 2.

9. *Ibid.*, p. 2.

10. P. Collins, *Dictionary of Scottish
    Business*, p. 104.

11. G.M. Shanks, p. 2.

12. Patent 1866/2183, p. 72. Jennings
    also made this closet with cylinders
    and traps of galvanised iron; see his
    advertisement in *The Ironmonger*
    supplement, 29 April 1881.

13. *The Builder*, 5 October 1878,
    p. 1048.

14. J. Bailey Denton, *Sanitary
    Engineering*, 1876, pp. 77–8.

15. *The Ironmonger*, 2 February 1874,
    p. 58, patent 1874/1175.

16. S. Stevens Hellyer, 1891, p. 207.

17. R. Palmer, p. 46.

18. Patent 1862/2286, G. White,
    F. Buckland and C. Rees for a
    wash-out closet and patent
    1866/1552, D.A. Dumius and
    others, p. 70.

19. Hellyer, 1877, p. 85.

20. Patent 1875/649, S.H. Rowley.

21. James Woodward claimed the name
    'wash-out' as a registered
    trademark, registered under the
    Trade Marks Act on 14 March
    1878, *The Ironmonger*, 16 August
    1884, p. 182.

22. Patent 1876/4424.

23. Hellyer, 1877, p. 86.

24. Patent 1877/1412.

25. Patent 1875//2801 and 1878/3114,
    J. Dodd, wash-out closets.

26. Hatton, p. 19.

27. The design of the 'Crown' was registered on 17 August 1882, Register of Designs, no. 6571 (PRO, BT 46/4).

28. T. Twyford, *Catalogue of Earthenware Sanitary Goods*, April 1883, p. 32.

29. R.K. Henrywood, *Bristol Potters 1775–1906*, Redcliffe, Bristol, 1992, p. 42.

30. *The Builder*, 25 October 1879, p. 1180.

31. *The Builder*, 1 November 1879, p. 1198.

32. These commendations were used by Woodward and Rowley to advertise their wash-out closet, *The Ironmonger*, 16 August 1884, p. 182.

33. *The Builder*, 31 May 1884, pp. 809–10, 7 June, pp. 846–7, 14 June, pp. 880–1, 21 June, pp. 916–7, 28 June, pp. 950–1.

34. *The Ironmonger*, 26 January, 1884, p. 51.

35. *The Builder*, 21 June 1884, p. 916.

36. *The Builder*, 21 June 1884, p. 917.

37. Hatton, p. 19.

38. The 'Florentine' design was registered on 28 August 1886, Register of Designs, no. 55420, (PRO, BT 50/71 and BT 51/28, p. 183).

39. The 'Dolphin' was registered on 31 December 1884, Register of Designs, no. 19753 (PRO, BT 50/25 and BT 51/10, p. 273).

40. *The Builder*, 25 September 1886, p. 465. From 1878, J. Dimmock and Co. was under the proprietorship of W.D. Cliff (i.e. Walter Cliff of Joseph Cliff and Sons), G.A. Godden, *Encyclopaedia of Pottery and Porcelain Marks*, 1964 edn, p. 208.

41. *Water Log, Federation Européenne des Fabricants de Ceramiques Sanitaires*, Darwin Finlayson, Chichester, n.d., p. 46. I am grateful to Simon Kirby for this reference.

42. Patent 1886/14,322, J. Smeaton. This patent refers to hopper basins, but by 1892 the Amphora shape was also available as a wash-out or valve closet, *The Ironmonger*, 2 January 1892, p. 36.

43. *The Ironmonger*, 2 January 1892, p. 36.

44. *The Health Journal*, August 1886, p. 44.

45. *The Builder*, 21 June 1884, p. 917.

46. *The Ironmonger*, 7 April 1888, p. lxi.

47. Hellyer, p. 220.

48. *Ibid.*, pp. 201–3.

49. *Ibid.*, p. 205.

50. *The Builder*, 26 September 1885, p. 423. It is possible, of course, that in giving higher awards to earth closets that the judges were pursuing their own agenda – that is, supporting the dry system of disposal.

51. F. Celoria, *Water Closets, Past, Present and Future*, 1981, p. 8 shows wash-down closets of a type being recommended in London in the late 1840s.

52. See, for example, the patents of S. Stocker, 1855/1639 and W. Phillips, 1875/984. W. Buchan's patent was 1879/5272.

53. Hellyer, 1877, p. 82.

54. Thomas Twyford catalogue, March 1879, p. 23. The 'Lillyman' closet is actually described as a washdown closet in Twyford's 1889 catalogue.

55. Hellyer, p. 82.

56. The design of this closet was registered on 16 March 1885. Register of Designs, no. 23738, (PRO BT50/30 and BT 51/12, p. 368). T. and W. Farmiloe catalogue, London, January 1886, pp. 46–7.

57. Hatton, p. 20.

58. Patent 1855/2091, p. 4.

59. *The Builder*, 9 January 1886, p. 70 and Plumbing World.com from an article first published in *P and M Magazine*, July 1994.

60. J. Shanks, patent 1894/6085.

61. T.W. Twyford, patent 1894/13,292.

62. S. Jennings, and J. Morley, patent 1894/13,782.

63. William Howell eliminated the lower trap of syphonic closets in 1890, *P and M Magazine*, July 1994.

64. *The Builder*, 9 January 1886, p. 70.

65. J.L. Mott Iron Works, New York, catalogue, 1888, reprinted by Dover Publications, New York, 1987, pp. 54, 69.

66. Information from Plumbing World.com from an article published in *P and M Magazine*, July 1994. See also Munroe Blair, *Ceramic Water Closets*, Shire, 2000, p. 30.

67. British Standards Institution, Ceramic Washdown WC. Pans, Dimensions and Workmanship, British Standard 1213:1945.

Chapter Eight

1. *The Builder*, 1 June 1878, p. 556.

2. H. Mayhew, *London Labour and the London Poor*, 1861, pp. 168–73.

3. W. Reyburn, *Flushed with Pride: The Story of Thomas Crapper*, 1969, p. 15.

4. H.B. King, *Water: The Book*, Quiller Press, 1992, p. 117.

5. D. Cruickshank and N. Burton, *Life in the Georgian City*, Viking Penguin, London, 1990, p. 96.

6. Bath Reference Library.

7. H.B. King, p. 117.

8. W.P. Buchan, *Plumbing*, 1876, pp. 169–71.

9. H.B. King, pp. 119–20.

10. F.C. Jones, *Bristol's Water Supply and its Story*, Bristol Waterworks Co., Bristol, 1946, p. 23.

11. In 1884 the number of supplies to houses in London was 668,525, but the number of houses on a constant supply was only 254,920. *The Iron-monger*, 16 August 1884, p. 204.

12. A. Briggs, *Victorian Cities*, 1963 and 1968, p. 324.

13. *Ibid.*, p. 224.

14. Quoted in R. Palmer, p. 92.

15. Buchan, p. 171.

16. Sir John Vanbrugh's Designs for Kings Weston, BRO 33746.

17. R. Palmer, p. 93.

18. J.H. Walsh, *Manual of Domestic Economy*, 1867, p. 62.

19. Patent, 8 March 1852/14001, F.G. Underhay.

20. These were displayed at the International Exhibition, London in 1862, catalogue, class X. p. 54.

21. Patent 1864/2061, G.F. Underhay and R. Heyworth.

22. Described by J. Bailey Denton, p. 83.

23. International Exhibition Catalogue, p. 54.

24. Warner and Sons catalogue, 1856, p. 50.

25. Patent 1856/1572, R.L. Howard.

26. Patent 1858/1500, J.G. Jennings and patent 1859/642, A. Tylor.

27. J. Bailey Denton, pp. 75–83 and patent 1873/907, A. Tylor.

28. Warner, p. 48.

29. Walsh, pp. 62–3 and patent 1854/1017, J.G. Jennings.

30. J. Bailey Denton, p. 88.

31. *Ibid.*, p. 86.

32. Patent 1854/1017, J.G. Jennings.

33. Patent 1874/1207, S. Peters and W. Donald.

34. The syphon became the only legal flushing device in Britain until 2000, when, due to pressure from the EU, valve cisterns were once again legalised.

35. *The Ironmonger*, 5 January 1884, p. 99.

36. *Ibid.*, 5 January 1884, p. 29.

37. S. Stevens Hellyer, *The Plumber and Sanitary Houses*, 1877, p. 130.

38. *The Ironmonger*, 15 March 1884, advertisements. This cistern was the subject of patent 1882/5885 by W.A.G. Schonheyder.

39. *Ibid.*, 12 July 1884, p. 47.

40. *Ibid.*, 23 November 1889, p. xliii.

41. *Ibid.*, 9 February 1884, p. 185 and 5 October 1889, p. xxx.

42. *Ibid.*, 23 November 1889, p. xliii.
43. Shanks and Co. catalogue, 1904, p. 393.
44. G.M. Shanks, *The First Hundred Years*, 1951, pp. 14–15. Shanks shipped 15,000 cisterns to Argentina in 1909 and 22,000 in 1910.
45. Shanks and Co., catalogue, 1893, pp. 200 and 203.
46. Patent 1796/2111, W. Law.
47. J.C. Loudon, *Cottage, Farm and Villa Architecture*, 1833, p. 150.
48. See, ch. 2, n. 2.
49. Patent 1887/3431, J. Duckett.
50. *The Builder*, 1 October 1887, p. 455.
51. *Ibid.*, 8 October 1887, p. 512.
52. See, for example, patents

1896/9407 and 1896/16,676, J. Duckett.
53. Patent 1892/17,728, J. Duckett.
54. Mavis Walton, née Eveleigh, b. 1919, Bradford.
55. Thus Thomas Crapper introduced a WWP fitted with a 'tranquil pipe' to deaden the noise of the cistern filling, in 1887, *The Builder*, 8 October 1887, p. 516. They fitted an air pipe to gradually end the emptying by syphonage to their 'Silent' WWP, E.G., Blake, *Plumbing: A Text-book to the Art or Craft of the Plumber*, 1948, p. 141.
56. Shanks's catalogue, 1893, p. 191.
57. Doulton and Co. catalogue, 1904, p. 37.

Chapter Nine

1. First Report of the Health of Towns Commission, vol. 2, p. 31, quoted in R.A. Lewis, *Edwin Chadwick and the Public Health Movement 1832–1854*, 1952, p. 92.
2. *Ibid.*, p. 42, quoting Chadwick to F.O. Ward, 7 October 1849.
3. J. Burnett, *A Social History of Housing*, 1978, pp. 184–6.
4. My own searches through building plans in Bristol suggest the bathroom was generally adopted in larger houses by *c.* 1880 (building plans, Bristol Record Office).
5. 'The Housing of the Agricultural Labourer', *JRASE*, vol. 75, 1914, p. 28.
6. G. Orwell, *The Road to Wigan Pier*, Gollancz, 1937 and Penguin, 1962, p. 34.
7. *Cassell's Household Guide*, *c.* 1869, p. 46.
8. E. Grey, p. 50.
9. E.C. Kitson, *Sanitary Lessons to Working Women in Leeds during the Winters of 1872 and 1873*, Ladies Council of the Yorkshire Board of Education, Leeds, 1873, p. 13.
10. G. Orwell, pp. 33–4.
11. W. Savage cites Dr H.J. Hunter's 'Report into the State of the

Dwellings of the Rural Poor', 1866, which found that out of a sample of 5,375 cottages, 40.8 per cent had only one bedroom, Savage, p. 20.
12. Orwell, p. 33.
13. F. Thompson, *Lark Rise to Candleford*, 1945 and Penguin 1973, p. 125.
14. *Ibid.*, pp. 431–2.
15. L. Levi, *Wages and Earnings of the Working Classes*, Report to Sir Arthur Bass, 1885, p. 30, quoted in J. Burnett, *Plenty and Want*, Nelson, 1966 and 1979, p. 127.
16. F. Thompson, p. 126.
17. Information supplied to the author by a former St Jude's slum dweller, Bristol, in the 1930s.
18. J. Somerville, *Christopher Thomas, Soapmaker of Bristol*, Redcliffe, Bristol, 1991, pp. 40–2.
19. 720 houses were built at Port Sunlight from 1888 and both the two main types of house contained bathrooms, Burnett, pp. 178–9. Bathrooms were also provided in houses on Cadbury's Bournville estate by *c.* 1900.
20. W.H. Fisher, *The Coming of the Mass Market, 1850–1914*,

Macmillan, 1981, pp. 53, 120, 205–6.

21. Kitson, p. 13.

22. The Royal School Series, *Domestic Economy: a Class Book for Girls*, T. Nelson, London, 1877, pp. 77–8, 102.

23. 'The Liverpool Health of Towns', *Advocate*, 15, 2 November 1846.

24. S. Sheard, *Profit is a Dirty Word: The Development of Public Baths and Wash Houses in Britain 1847–1915*, The Society for the Social History of Medicine, 2000, p. 68.

25. *The Builder*, 6 June 1878, p. 706.

26. G. Orwell, p. 61.

27. D. Jones, *Counting the Cost of Coal*, p. 116.

28. The 1923 catalogue of Gardiner and Sons, wholesale ironmongers, Bristol, contained three styles of hip baths.

29. R.A. Church, *Kenricks in Hardware*, p. 179.

30. *Ibid*.

31. R.L. Blaszczyk, *Imagining Consumers, Design and Innovation from Wedgwood to Corning*, Johns Hopkins University Press, Baltimore and London, 2000, p. 168.

32. *Ibid.*, p. 199.

33. Rowe Brothers and Co., catalogue 90, 1939, p. 5.

34. Blaszczyk, p. 199.

35. M. and N. Ward, *Home in the Twenties and Thirties*, Ian Allan, 1978, pp. 84–5.

36. *The Ironmonger*, 'Bathroom Number', 22 April 1939, p. 94.

37. *Ibid.*, p. 92. Bert Hodgkiss, who worked for Twyford's for over fifty years, recalls that repairing scratched toilet seats kept their two French polishers busy and was a lucrative business for the company.

38. *Ibid.*, 2 April 1939, p. 94.

39. I am indebted to Terry Wooliscroft of Twyford's for drawing these dates in the company's own records to my attention.

40. F. de Bonneville, *The Book of the Bath*, 1997, p. 135.

41. W.G. Walker, *Sanitary Pottery*, 1924, p. 13.

Bibliography

Books

Atterbury, P. and Irvine, L., *The Doulton Story*, Royal Doulton Tableware, Stoke-on-Trent, 1979

Ayres, J., *Building the Georgian City*, Yale, New Haven and London, 1998

Barty King, H., *Water: The Book*, Quiller Press, 1992

Binding, H., *Somerset Privies*, Countryside Books, Newbury, Berkshire, 1999

Binnie, R. and Boxall, J., *Household Principles and Practice*, Pitman, London, n.d., c. 1930

Blake, E.G., *Plumbing: A Text-book to the Art or Craft of the Plumber*, The Technical Press, London, 4th ed., 1948

Blair, M., *Ceramic Water Closets*, Shire, Princes Risborough, 2000

Blair, M., *Bathroom Ceramics*, Shire, Princes Risborough, 2002

de Bonneville, F., *The Book of the Bath*, Flammarion Press, Paris, trans. Jane Brenton, Thames and Hudson, London, 1998

Blaszczyk, R. Lee, *Imagining Consumers, Design and Innovation from Wedgwood to Corning*, Johns Hopkins University Press, Baltimore and London, 2000

Briggs, A., *Victorian Cities*, Odhams Press, 1963 and Penguin, 1968

Briggs, A., *Victorian Things*, Batsford, London, 1988

Buchan, W.P., *Plumbing*, Crosby Lockwood and Co., London, 1876

Burnett, J., *A Social History of Housing, 1815–1970*, David and Charles, Newton Abbot, 1978

Cassell's Household Guide, London, 1869–71

Celoria, F., *Water Closets, Past, Present and Future*, Gladstone Pottery Museum, Stoke-on-Trent, 1981

Clow, G.B., *Practical Up-to-Date Plumbing*, Frederick J. Drake, Chicago, 1906 and 1914

Cruickshank, D. and Burton, N., *Life in the Georgian City*, Viking Penguin, London, 1990

Denton, J.B., *Sanitary Engineering*, Spon, London, 1877

Donno, E. Story, *Sir John Harington's A New Discourse on a Stale Subject called the Metamorphosis of Ajax*, Routledge and Kegan Paul, London, 1962

Eassie, W., *Sanitary Arrangements for Dwellings*, South Elder, London, 1874

Forty, A., *Objects of Desire – Design and Society 1750–1980*, Thames and London, 1986

Gavin, H., *Sanitary Ramblings*, John Churchill, London, 1848

Girouard, M., *Life in the English Country House*, Yale, New Haven and London, 1978

Graham, F., *The Geordie Netty*, Northern History Booklet, Newcastle-upon-Tyne, 1977

Halliday, S., *The Great Stink of London*, Sutton Publishing, Stroud, 1999

Hall, L., *Down the Garden Path*, Countryside Books, Newbury, 2001

Harris, M., *Cotswold Privies*, Chatto and Windus, London, 1984

Hart-Davies, A., *Thunder, Flush and Thomas Crapper*, Michael O'Mara Books, London, 1997

Hatton, J., *Twyfords: A Century in the History of Potters*, J.S. Virtue, London, 1905

Hellyer, S. Stevens, *The Plumber and Sanitary Houses*, Batsford, London, 1877

Hellyer, S. Stevens, *Lectures on the Science and Art of Sanitary Plumbing*, Batsford, London, 1882

Hellyer, S. Stevens, *Principles and Practice of Plumbing, George Bell and Sons*, London, 1891

Hogg, J., *London As It Is*, Mitcham, London, 1837

Hole, J., *The Homes of the Working Classes*, Longman, Green and Co., London, 1866

Horan, J.L., *The Porcelain God, A Social History of the Toilet*, Carol Publishing Group, New Jersey, 1996

Jephson, H., *The Sanitary Evolution of London*, Fisher Unwin, London, 1907

Lambton, L., *Temples of Convenience*, Gordon Fraser, London, 1978

Lambton, L., *Temples of Convenience and Chambers of Delight*, Pavilion, London, 1995

Lewis, D., *Kent Privies*, Countryside Books, Newbury, 1996

Lewis, R.A., *Edwin Chadwick and the Public Health Movement 1832–1854*, Longman, Green and Co., 1952

Loudon, J.C., *Cottage Farm and Villa Architecture*, Longman, London, 1833

McLaughlin, T., *Coprophilia or a Peck of Dirt*, Cassell, 1971

McNeil, I., *Joseph Bramah, A Century of Invention*, David and Charles, Newton Abbot, 1968

Markham, L., *Yorkshire Privies*, Countryside Books, Newbury, 1996

Mayhew, H., *London Labour and the London Poor*, Griffin, London, 1851 and 1861–2

Murphy, S. Forster, *Our Homes and How to Make Them Healthy*, Cassell, London, 1883

Muthesius, H., *The English House*, Berlin, 1904/5, trans. Janet Seligman, Crosby, Lockwood Staples, London, 1979

Muthesius, S., *The English Terraced House*, Yale University Press, New Haven and London, 1982

Palmer, R., *The Water Closet, A New History*, David and Charles, Newton Abbot, 1973

Newbold, H. Bryant, *House and Cottage Construction*, chs by Martin, A.C., 'Sanitary Plumbing and Waste Disposal Work', Caxton, London, n.d., *c*. 1930

Reyburn, W., *Flushed with Pride, The Story of Thomas Crapper*, Macdonald and Co., 1969 and Pavilion Books, London, 1989

Roberts, J.A., *North Wales Privies*, Countryside Books, Newbury, 1998

Rolt, L.T.C., *Victorian Engineering*, Penguin, 1970

Sale, C., *The Specialist*, Putnam and Co., London, 1930

Savage, W.G., *Rural Housing*, Fisher Unwin, London, 1915

Scott, G. Ryley, *The Story of Baths and Bathing*, T. Werner Laurie Ltd, 1939

Shanks, G.M., *The First Hundred Years 1851–1951*, Shanks, Barrhead, n.d., *c*. 1951

Spavold, J., *The Sanitary Pottery Industries of South Derbyshire, 1840–1914*, MSc Thesis, UMIST, Faculty of Science and Technology, 1978

Taine, H., *Notes on England*, Strahan, London, 1872

Teale, T. Pridgin, *Dangers to Health. A Pictorial Guide to Sanitary Defects*, J. and A. Churchill, London, 1879

Thornton, P., *Authentic Décor. The Domestic Interior 1620–1920*, Weidenfeld and Nicolson, 1984

Thompson, F., *Lark Rise to Candleford*, Oxford University Press, 1945, Penguin, 1973

Turner, J., *East Anglian Privies*, Countryside Books, Newbury, 1995

Vacher, F., *Defects in Plumbing and Drainage Work*, J. Heywood, Manchester and London, 1889

Walker, W.G., *Sanitary Pottery*, Twyfords, Hanley, 1924

Walsh, J.H., *A Manual of Domestic Economy*, G. Routledge, London, 1857

Ward, T., *Henry Moule of Fordington 1801–1880. Radical Parson and Inventor*, E.W. Ward, Poole, Dorset, n.d.

Webster, T., *An Encyclopaedia of Domestic Economy*, Longman, London, 1844

Wedd, K., *The Victorian Bathroom Catalogue*, Studio Editions, 1996

Wilson, G., *A Handbook of Hygiene*, J. and A. Churchill, London, 1873

Woodcroft, B., *Alphabetical Index of Patentees of Inventions*, 1854 and Evelyn, Adams and Mackay, London, 1969

Wright, L., *Clean and Decent*, Routledge and Kegan Paul, London, 1960

Trade Catalogues

Baxendale and Co., Manchester, *c.* 1902

Broad and Co., Paddington, 1910

Thomas Crapper and Co., Chelsea, 1888

Doulton and Co., Lambeth etc., various dates

T. and W. Farmiloe, London,1886

Gardiner Sons and Co., Bristol, various dates

Hampton and Sons, London,1894

Humpherson and Co., Chelsea, 1887

George Jennings, Stangate, various dates

Richard Johnson, Liverpool and Manchester, 1902

John Jones, Chelsea, 1906

Llewellins and James, Bristol, 1889

McFarlane's Castings, Glasgow, *c.* 1880

Metal Agencies Co., Bristol, various dates

Milton, Falkirk and Glasgow, *c.* 1906

Morrison, Ingram and Co., Manchester, *c.* 1893

The J.L Mott Iron Works, New York and Chicago, 1888, reprint

Pountney and Co., Bristol, various dates

The Reading Iron Company, 1910

Rowe Brothers, Exeter and Bristol, various dates

Shanks and Co., Barrhead, various dates

Sharpe Brothers and Co., Swadlincote

Thomas W. Twyford and later Twyford catalogues, Hanley, various dates

John Warner and Sons, Cripplegate, London, 1856

Index